Routledge Revivals

MINDS IN DISTRESS

MINDS IN DISTRESS

A PSYCHOLOGICAL STUDY OF THE MASCULINE AND FEMININE MIND IN HEALTH AND IN DISORDER

BY

A. E. BRIDGER

B.A., B.Sc, M.D., F.R.S. (EDIN.)

Fellow of the Royal College of Physicians of Edinburgh ; Fellow of the
Royal Society of Medicine of London

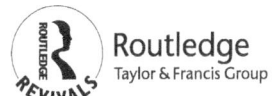

First published in 1913 by Methuen & Co. Ltd.

This edition first published in 2018 by Routledge
2 Park Square, Milton Park, Abingdon, Oxon, OX14 4RN
and by Routledge
711 Third Avenue, New York, NY 10017

Routledge is an imprint of the Taylor & Francis Group, an informa business

© 1913 Taylor & Francis

All rights reserved. No part of this book may be reprinted or reproduced or utilised in any form or by any electronic, mechanical, or other means, now known or hereafter invented, including photocopying and recording, or in any information storage or retrieval system, without permission in writing from the publishers.

Publisher's Note
The publisher has gone to great lengths to ensure the quality of this reprint but points out that some imperfections in the original copies may be apparent.

Disclaimer
The publisher has made every effort to trace copyright holders and welcomes correspondence from those they have been unable to contact.
A Library of Congress record exists under ISBN.

ISBN 13: 978-1-138-55261-6 (hbk)
ISBN 13: 978-1-138-56882-2 (pbk)
ISBN 13: 978-0-203-70473-8 (ebk)

MINDS IN DISTRESS

BY THE SAME AUTHOR

MAN AND HIS MALADIES
THE TREATMENT OF CONSUMPTION
DYSPEPSIA PERFECT AND IMPERFECT
DEPRESSION, ETC.

MINDS IN DISTRESS

A PSYCHOLOGICAL STUDY OF THE MASCULINE AND FEMININE MIND IN HEALTH AND IN DISORDER

BY

A. E. BRIDGER

B.A., B.Sc., M.D., F.R.S. (EDIN.)

Fellow of the Royal College of Physicians of Edinburgh; Fellow of the Royal Society of Medicine of London

METHUEN & CO. LTD.
36 ESSEX STREET W.C.
LONDON

First Published in 1913

PREFACE

THERE are two points from which humanity may be viewed, the bodily and the mental.

Hitherto, and for various reasons, medicine has concerned itself almost solely with the physical side of man.

The result has been disappointing, for, necessary as it is to be acquainted with the bodily structure in health and in disease, the changes that occur in the latter only represent the physical results of a process, and not the means by which the damage is done.

Now the duty of the physician is like that of the pilot; to bring his patient safely into port, availing himself of every agency with that one object in view.

Therefore, Mind, in the fullest and widest sense, must be one of his chief studies.

But the subject, when we try to confine it within rules, presents great and special difficulties, and only principles that are of universal acceptance, free of speculative theory and reducible to the simplest terms, are likely to be of any practical utility.

Of these, I formulate two: 1st, That mental comfort depends on a state of balance between two main factors in the human mind. 2nd, That all minds are divisible into two great types according as the reasoning or the instinctive faculties predominate. I call them, respectively, the masculine and feminine types of mind. I avoid the words male and female, since the line of division is not one solely dependent on sex.

In the following pages I shall define the above propositions, and show that upon them depend the functional nervous disorders that afflict humanity, the obscurity of whose origin is attested by the great variety of names, *e.g.*, Neurasthenia, Psychasthenia, Hysteria, Hypochondriasis,

PREFACE

Neuroses, etc., etc., under which the text-books treat of them.

As my appeal is one to the common experience of humanity I shall make use of the simplest language at my command, and as my thesis is—as far as I know—an entirely novel one, I shall not refer to well-known writers on the subject as they all approach it from an entirely different point of view.

Foley Lodge,
  5 Langham Street,
    Portland Place,
      London, W.

CONTENTS

CHAP.		PAGE
I.	THE NORMAL MIND AND MENTAL BALANCE	1
II.	THE MASCULINE TYPE OF MIND	17
III.	THE FEMININE TYPE OF MIND	24
IV.	NEURASTHENIA	37
V.	THE TREATMENT, ETC., OF NEURASTHENIA	59
VI.	HYSTERIA	81
VII.	HYSTERIA	108
VIII.	HYSTERIA	128
IX.	MENTAL FORMULÆ	168
	INDEX	179

"Das ist's ja was den Menschen zieret,
Und dazu ward ihm der Verstand,
Das er im innern Herzen spüret
Was er erschafft mit seiner Hand."

SCHILLER

MINDS IN DISTRESS

CHAPTER I

THE NORMAL MIND AND MENTAL BALANCE

WE must first get a clear and concise *general* idea of Mind.

Many of my readers probably have read the shorter treatises on Psychology by William James, Titchener, Wundt and others. If so, they will have been struck, as I have, by the fact that, when dealing with detached and strictly physiological problems, such as can easily be verified by experiment, the writers are much at home, but that when these have been exhausted, and the stage of generalization has been reached, when the reader is on the tiptoe of expectation, eager for a new and cogent definition of Mind as a going process, the author becomes vague and drifts away into a discussion on Monism, Atomism, Occasionalism, Spiritualism, etc.; in short, he

trembles, so to speak, on the confines of Metaphysics, and there he perforce leaves us.

And the reason for this is simple. Body and mind are one and indivisible, but two views of the same entity.

Keep as conscientiously as you may to the physiological, the biochemical and the mechanical, reject every proposition that is not valid in science, yet you come inevitably to a wall, more solid and repellent the stricter you have been with yourself, which bars all further progress, and have to acknowledge with Karl Pearson in his admirable *Grammar of Science* that the search for ultimate truth on scientific lines leads but eventually to self-contradiction. You start with X as representing the unknown, the vital or the psyche; you work on and seem to get fair representation values in physiology for certain components of X, but you never reach a solution, change your method as you may. Only on the material side are you happy, for with so many data in hand, and such an army of skilled collaborating investigators, you instinctively feel that, in a sensible future, nearly every tissue and function will be

THE NORMAL MIND

ranged and measured, and the body of man, as *stationary and inert, fixed in time and space*, will come to be represented by a chemico-mechanical formula of great complexity but of definite accuracy, and that, as a final triumph, you may even reasonably expect a day when there will be made a synthetic protoplasm that shall live.

But that will not have solved the problem. You will only have supplied a further instance of what we all know, that when Mind demands anything imperatively, out somewhere from the environment comes tissue to clothe the idea, to give it what we call a material basis, to do, in short, what evolution—whether consciously or not, who shall decide?—has been doing down all the ages and what she is doing daily in the field of physiology, not only by adding and developing new function and tailoring it, but by causing to degenerate and disappear that for which she has no present use. You will have given further proof that Mind, whether represented in the person of modern man armed with weapons of precision, or as a vague creative force omnipresent in all that we call nature, is the great generator,

the real *causa causans*, and that matter is ever an obedient servant that faithfully carries out her commands.

You will have made life and mind. No; you will have made both possible. A great achievement indeed in the popular view though the idea that a great barrier divides the living from the non-living is a purely arbitrary one. None of the roads leads to a real conception of mind in its essence. We measure the force and rate of certain minor functions of the brain, those of the special senses in particular which lend themselves to the process readily, and we work unremittingly onwards to a more intimate knowledge of the cell structure through which mind acts, but only to find the mystery deepening and to realize the enormous gap that exists in this matter between knowledge and understanding.

To obtain any useful basis from which to classify and study mind we have to depend on certain anatomical and physiological facts just as far as they carry us and then to study these in the light of wide experience. Only thus shall we find practical guides in our work and obtain any useful general rule

THE NORMAL MIND 5

that will command the acceptance of all thoughtful men.

The Human Mind.—This is best classified according to its duties into three great parts: the conscious, the subconscious and the reflex, automatic or organic. Acting all together as in normal persons they constitute the *Ego*. But they must *not be thought of as separate* except as a matter of convenience in speaking. True, in the average life of man each keeps its place in function, and we thus come to view them as distinct; but *there are no fixed and real boundaries*, and directly circumstances become unusual the order of this relationship is overthrown and they invade each other's department and provide us with many extraordinary phenomena. Some minds, being more active than others, or proportioned differently, show this intermingling of function early and under slight stress, and in them—as we shall see—it may reach easily a great development, and indeed with a little trouble, and by arranging our environment, we can induce artificially, and even in persons who are in the enjoyment of normal health, many of these abnormal

phenomena as we see in hypnotism and spiritualism.

This contiguity—this close relationship—throughout the body of the three great departments of mind is a matter of importance and must be kept in view, and though we speak anatomically of "mapped-out areas of the brain," and of the "great special centres" therein, we do this largely as a matter of convenience, for it is not even certain that within the brain reside all the functions of thought; and Dr Charlton Bastian, amongst other authorities, holds that the great ganglia of the sympathetic system, which are chiefly in the abdomen, "have a large share in the conscious life of the individual and lead more or less directly to a series of voluntary actions," whilst the most extensive and destructive disease in the brain, as subsequently viewed in post-mortems, has been present with a practically unimpaired intellect of the sufferer. It is therefore safer to keep in mind the three great mental departments without tying these down at all strictly to special areas in the brain.

At present the conscious department

THE NORMAL MIND

alone concerns us and we shall deal with it on the broadest principles of experience.

Mental Balance.—One arm of this balance is what we may call *Common Sense*. This consists of our general store of knowledge, a register of our conclusions to date, and though it is being perpetually modified in composition by such new ideas as we accept and absorb, yet is the more stable arm of the balance. It is constantly being kept in a state of *general average* with other minds by means of contact with the current opinion of the day, a point that is of great practical importance in life, for when an individual, or even a whole group of persons, as in a profession, isolates himself and fails to keep in touch with the world in general, he is in great danger of mental distress, for his standard is lost and with it his sense of proportion. This is one of the great causes of many mental and nervous disorders.

The other arm of the balance, for so we must call it, is made up of the *new* impressions which in countless variety and from all sources, from our internal organs and from the outside world, reach and are presented to the common sense as to a standard. If

the latter be kept active and well stored by incessant readjustment with the world-mind, and if the nerve tissue on which mind rests as its material basis be healthy and adaptable, very rarely indeed will any fresh impression remain unbalanced, but unnoticed, and I may say almost automatically, find a place in and become a part of the common sense, while even if the new circumstance with its impressions cannot be thus at once and directly assimilated it will create no disorder, for the mind will "throw out a balance," as it is called in philosophic language, will adopt a theory that will for the time being bring the two arms of the balance into equilibrium. This state is called "making up one's mind."

Now all this may appear too commonplace to require formal statement, yet on this balancing of the two factors—the normal impression with the common sense—mental comfort depends, and from a want of it far-reaching mental distress arises.

Note how much depends on the soundness and stability of the common sense. If all minds were compounded in exactly similar proportions of the three constituent parts—

THE NORMAL MIND

the conscious, subconscious and automatic—if all nerve tissue were always in a state of similar activity, and if the environment of everyone were equally restricted and exactly alike, then, at least at equal ages, people would all possess an equal common sense, and any serious difficulty from the failure to reach a balance could rarely arise; but there is a wide variation in all the above factors, and consequently an enormous difference in the response to unusual or novel sensations; and the result of this failure to reach an equilibrium is to give rise to phenomena of disorder altogether incomprehensible to persons of different mental capacity and to the world at large, and leads to grave misunderstanding, the failure to balance being wrongly ascribed to some vague agent of disease attacking the body from without, when all the time it is due simply to the fact that the mind (the common sense) of the patient is of different composition to that of the observer and is merely responding in a way normal to itself.

For that reason it is essential to closely study the *mental composition* of the sufferer

from mental distress so as to be able to interpret the symptoms observed, which will usually be found to be only natural under the circumstances and not due to some supposed malignant external agency. Then by effecting a change in the environment, by adapting the latter as closely as possible to the individual needs and requirements, health may often be easily restored, and measures having been taken to effect a constant healthy contact of the sufferer with the general world-mind, a stable and lasting condition of mental comfort under all ordinary circumstances of life may be secured. Therefore the very simple, elementary balance of which I have spoken must ever be kept in mind.

Now, in the event of novel experience, the throwing out of a balance by the mind to effect an equilibrium in the person of good sound common sense, who lives in free contact with the world-mind, is a simple process leading to no distress. The provisional theory adopted is either affirmed by experience, or if not, the theory is rejected and another conformable to general ideas

THE NORMAL MIND

is adopted. But when the common sense is not of an average and sound order, by reason of the isolation in life of its possessor, or because his mental composition is not in the usually relative proportions, or when the mind is of extreme sensitiveness by inheritance, impressions quite ordinary of their kind and easily balanced in the former may lead in the latter to the adoption of a theory that, while it appears quite right to the individual, is widely at variance with the ordinary world-mind of the day, and for that reason—even independently of isolation—be extremely difficult to correct. Of this nature are the so-called "Obsessions" and "Phobias" of the Neurasthenic, the grievances to which some persons seem so pertinaciously to cling and the distorted views of the Hysterical. These appear weird and unreal to the man of the world, or even as evidence of a diseased mind, whereas, when all the circumstances of the case are known, they are easily seen to have had a simple origin and to be natural theories, efforts made by a common sense for some reason out of touch with the ordinary mind of the day

but perfectly sound, though often highly sensitive.

These wandering ghosts of ideas that have thus taken their rise, these theories formed naturally to effect a mental balance, become in time accepted more or less as real, and, instead of being corrected by a common sense in contact with the living moving world, themselves become so uppermost in the mind as to pervert it; so that you get the picture of a man who is strictly sane, and indeed very logical, but all whose arguments, with the consequences that flow from them, are founded on an initial theory which he has never been able to displace, and which has grown and blossomed by isolation and introspection. He has been the victim of self-suggestion, of a *disorder of the attention*, and can only be cured, as we shall see, by one who will completely unravel the tangle and at the same time place and keep the sufferer in the active, moving world of normal minds.

The aforesaid process has nothing in common with the genesis of the Insane mind; the latter is generally due to a poisoning of the brain tissue by some failure in the de-

THE NORMAL MIND

fensive powers of the body and the consequent absorption into the blood of poisons generated usually in the bowel. In fact the brain, like the rest of the body, is singularly tolerant of mere mishandling such as occurs in the cases I have sketched, and organic disease is a most unusual consequence thereof, though degeneration may, in later life, be one of the sequences. Thus it happens that Neurasthenia and Hysteria, and other mere failures of mental balance, may be completely recovered from after a course of many years, and are indeed often automatically cured by the choice advent of some overmastering idea, especially by some very strong distressing experience.

Mental balance between the common sense (the formed individual conscious mind) and all novel experience that is presented to it thus means mental comfort, and the want of it mental distress that may, if favoured by circumstance, be of a most far-reaching kind.

Such, in the simplest of language, is the psychic basis from which mental suffering of a functional order takes its rise. The

symptoms that ensue depend, as to their character chiefly on the class of mind possessed by the patient, and as to their extent on his or her circumstances in life, especially as to a free or a restricted contact with other normal minds; the active world of working life being the great agent that moulds the human mind, the common sense, and maintains in it a healthy circulation of thought and that fits it for doing its best work.

The following simple illustrations will help to make clear my statements.

A. sees a ghostly figure at night. He knows that it is merely a shadow picture thrown by a magic-lantern and is unconcerned. Or he does not know of the magic-lantern and is upset. His friends persuade him that it is an optical delusion, and as he finds that these are fairly common he accepts the theory and is at rest. Or he cannot accept that theory, but regards the figure as the ghost of a departed friend sent as a warning, consults spiritualists, who advise a recourse to séances to clear up the mystery. He agrees and is soon in a state of advancing "abnormality."

THE NORMAL MIND 15

His common sense is being progressively perverted.

B., a bank clerk leading a routine life and therefore in mental isolation, has a sudden attack of depression with fear of loss of self-control. It is due to a cause unknown to him but really quite simple, an acute liver congestion. Instead of consulting a doctor, who would have told him that such attacks are quite common and what they arise from, and that a blue pill, a Turkish bath, a little care in diet, and an occasional game of golf, would correct matters and keep him free of such experiences, he adopts the theory of incipient insanity, and by reading up the latter subject persuades himself that he is right. He gets sick-leave and further isolates himself. The false theory is followed out logically in all directions and he becomes at last, by incessant thought on the subject, and by association with sympathizers, a miserable hypochondriac.

These examples make clear two facts of great importance, viz., that novel impressions which concern ourselves closely have a far greater effect than others in disturbing our mental comfort and balance, and that

isolation favours introspection and often leads to the adoption of a theory which appears to others out of all reasonable proportion to the symptoms, for the standard of the isolated man is a falsified one.

CHAPTER II

THE MASCULINE TYPE OF MIND

IN conversation about the ordinary affairs of life, and more especially in discussions on formal topics, whether of politics, ethics, or art in any form, you will remark that educated people may readily be divided into two main classes: the one very practical, who demand proof before they accept a conclusion and rely only on facts, evidently regarding a so-called fact as a final truth; the other class who live in a different plane of thought altogether, who assert that the effect will be so-and-so, who see the end to be attained and seem to be little concerned with the process by which it is reached, and much devoted to ideals. Among the former will be found the plodding, steady people who achieve financial success, or at least stability; among the latter the brilliant, artistic, creative and the spiritual. The genius is of the latter class.

Of course the dividing line between the two classes is not a hard-and-fast one; some have mental characteristics that are a blend of both types in various proportion. The first class is that endowed with the *Masculine* type of mind. Speaking generally the Englishman, the Lowland Scot and the North-Country Irishman are good specimen proofs of this order, and many even of their womenfolk are thus mentally constructed. Science in all its branches and business in all its forms are served by individuals of this type of mind, and legal and political affairs of necessity depend upon it.

It is the mind of the vast majority of men in this country. Without having studied formal logic they are logical and rely on the relation of cause and effect, considering that the one and only criterion of sane judgment. They can conceive of no other valid process of thought and utilize it alone in all their transactions and discussions.

Now what would you expect to find, if the balance of mind be disturbed in anyone of the masculine type? A series of reasoned

THE MASCULINE MIND

arguments as to their state. This is what you find in the Hypochondriacal type of Depression, the Neurasthenia of the textbooks. Throughout all his complaints the sufferer reasons and reasons.

Let me give an instance:

B., *æt.* forty, up to three years ago engaged in very routine office work in the Civil Service. Four years ago was attacked with dyspeptic symptoms and occasional sickness, followed later on by an irritating rash. Consulted advertisement in papers and medical books. Decided it was blood-poisoning of some most unusual kind for no doctor could give it a name. Searched his memory and thought that he must on one occasion have swallowed an infected blood clot. Advised a rest cure at first, and being unrelieved, gave up his work in order to devote his whole mind to his complaint. Attended hospitals diligently, and when I saw him was covered with sulphur ointment, which had induced very naturally a general state of eczema. He presented me with quite a treatise on his complaint. Founded on the theory of the blood clot he had built up by strict reasoning a whole

series of the consequences to be expected, and, partly by mental suggestion and partly by the absurd skin treatment given him by doctors sick of his loquacity, he had in part achieved most of them. The case looked unpromising for the whole mind was concentrated on self.

Though not strictly apropos, I will give the result. I accepted, provisionally, the theory of the blood clot, wrote my decided opinion that I could cure him, and, having ascertained what he would accept as proof thereof, got rid of the eczema, put him on a vegetarian diet, and insisted, before I would proceed further, on his return to work. He was taken back and given an active outdoor job by my advice. I gave him a mild subcutaneous injection of arsenic, which impressed him, and put him on his word of honour to consult no one, not even myself, and to read no medical book, for six months. The man is now in perfect health and quite sees how his former hypochondriasis was produced. But he maintains that without a definite written, closely-argued opinion and a written promise of complete cure, he would never have

THE MASCULINE MIND 21

succeeded in fighting his way out of the tangle.

F., a prosperous city merchant, came to tell me that he was becoming, if indeed he was not actually, insane. Why the theory of insanity? Because he was haunted with an idea so absurd that no practical and sane mind could harbour it. He had stolen a pot of jam thirty years ago, but had forgotten all about it, and this was the idea that had resurged in his mind and *would not go*. First of all I pointed out to him that the theft was a fact, not a delusion at all; that all his proofs of insanity, *i.e.*, some trifling loss of memory, extra sensitiveness, some sleeplessness, etc., are not complained of, though often present, in insanity and were evidently in his case induced by self-suggestion. Finally, that the memory of the theft was part of a train of thought induced by the words of a man in a heated discussion and who had said, "F., you were always a thief." Quite undeserved, this insult had rankled, and the word "*always*" was especially dwelt upon. I pointed out to him that every event of his past life he had recalled, balanced by his

mind and put to rest, but the idea of this one little theft, actual and real, never discovered and never forgiven, had remained behind, isolated and unbalanceable, and for that reason, and just because he was a just and conscientious man, the idea of this theft stood out prominently. It was simply a very sane idea.

It were easy to give instances innumerable, all with the same sequence. A novel idea or impression; a theory based thereon; long, logical arguments based on that theory, producing by their mental influence a series of symptoms, taken to be proofs of the theory; further arguments based on these false proofs, and the end a tangle of reasoning through which cause and effect, effect and cause, appear and reappear in every sentence; all the result of an active, sane, masculine type of mind struggling, by the only process it knows, to account to itself for a novel, and therefore disturbing, mental impression.

Yet the reader will see that two other influences have an effect on the result. The sufferer in the first case had not only the masculine type of mind but an abnormally active one, and his great mistake at the be-

ginning was to *isolate himself*, to settle down to think out, to discuss with himself, his theory. Had he but fortified his common sense by a more active communion with his fellow-men, had he thrown himself with greater fervour into work and taken on new forms of work, he would soon have recovered in one way or another his balance of mind and with it his mental composure.

And when we come to Neurasthenia we shall see that it is the specially active, the high-class, and therefore the naturally isolated, kind of masculine mind that usually falls a victim and why it is that so-called rest cures or abstention from work aggravate the evil by favouring that isolation, thus rendering more remote the chances of a speedy cure.

CHAPTER III

THE FEMININE TYPE OF MIND

THIS type is extremely difficult to describe. It is indeed inscrutable to its possessor. Its limits are not confined to what is usually styled the conscious brain. In addition to the reasoning faculty which it possesses in common with the masculine type, but upon which it by no means like the latter exclusively relies, it depends largely on intuition, on instinct, that, like the homing instincts of birds and animals, lead it aright across spaces that are apparently destitute of any guide or pathway. The vast majority of women have this class of mind, and we recognize in their deep instincts, such as that of maternity, in their unselfish love, in certain of their intuitive decisions, and in their quick insight into character, a faculty that guides them to a knowledge in which reason and experience play no part. Other and entirely non-

THE FEMININE MIND 25

sexual instincts are present in both men and women who are of this mental type, creative, decorative, imaginative, spiritual in kind. Genius is of this order. It is there, standing unsupported as it were and quite escaping the ring-fence of any verbal definition founded on cause and effect. It is said to be a gift, another word for instinct but not an explanation thereof. The great ideas that in history have moved mankind and swayed destinies are products of high-class feminine types of mind, and while in a region of ultimates, where there can exist no standards, one cannot accord priority of rank, yet one may legitimately entertain a "strong doubt" as to whether the feminine is not the higher. The two types are often said to be complementary one of the other, though there is not much sense or finality in the remark. But there it is, the type so common in all women, and in both sexes of the Latin and Celtic races, and its existence lies at the very root of the great differences of opinion — the *causa causans* of the wide chasm—that prevent a perfect understanding between peoples. The masculine and feminine types when in

different sexes blend admirably, but never in different nations who perpetually fail to do justice to each other's motives because of the mental medium by which alone they can judge being essentially different in colour.

What about this wider, deeper, feminine type of mind, this mind that does not depend solely on the grey matter of the brain as its basis but embraces the unconscious portions—and remember we have no right to rank either part as a higher one—when it loses balance?

Not the ordered argument, not the records of hours and days devoted to introspection, to a logical ordering of each section of a mental problem; not the reliance on cause and effect as with the masculine type, but an upheaval of wide extent, a volcanic eruption, a mingling of capricious thought and of disordered or convulsive action. That is what you would expect, that is what you get, and it is called Hysteria.

At this point again I must add, to avoid possible misunderstanding, that though, for the sake of clearness, I describe the two

THE FEMININE MIND

types of mind as widely separate yet in actual life they are often blended, scarcely ever perhaps in equal proportion; one type is usually recognizable as predominant but instances of pure type are by no means rare.

How does the great rule of mental balance affect the feminine type of mind? In the masculine type we had a comparatively simple problem that lent itself kindly to definition. Simple reason, as codified by formal logic and as applied every day in our business occupations and our scientific studies, in a state of distress, seeking by a fundamental rule of the mind to recover the balance of health and borrowing a counterbalance, *i.e.*, throwing out a theory, to that end, but often coming to grief by an excessive reliance on its own strong virtue, pure reason; the wanderer being further confused by the extravagant terms and theories of the guides to whom he applies for direction, like Sganarelle in his interview with Pancrace, doctor *in utroque jure*, in the "Mariage forcé" of Molière.

The feminine type of mind is, like the

masculine, and like every human mind, the result of a balance between the two parts thereof; an individual mind made up of impressions and ideas constantly being formed and a common mind (common sense) which represents the sum of acquired knowledge, plus certain instincts, the latter being the main element in the feminine type and which may be said to permeate it.

Under natural conditions, that is under such as afford scope for its full satisfaction and development, the feminine type of mind passes through life in a state of health. Its equilibrium is always a more delicate one than in the other type but small disturbances are rectified by the emotions acting as safety valves. How often do we not see a flow of tears in a woman or in a man of the Latin race bring relief to mental tension of the most varied kinds.

The disequilibration of the feminine type which we have later to study under the name of Hysteria varies of course as widely in its forms as the mind from which it has sprung, and will be seen to arise usually from two great causes—a repression of instincts and an exaggeration of self.

THE FEMININE MIND

Now instincts are never clear in consciousness. Take the maternal instinct: many women are never conscious of it, others feel it only as a vague impulse towards some end, and very few women ever devote serious thought to it, as they would to a problem in science. In civilized countries, where the masculine type of mind almost alone makes the laws and largely the social customs, all instincts have to be somewhat repressed, if they threaten to obtrude themselves unduly on public attention; for reasoning power must always have the most prominent position as controlling agent; and this is beneficial, for the mind, like the body, grows in strength as it grows in ordered self-control.

For if the bringing-up of a girl has been such that all the trivial cravings of the child mind for the indulgence of self have been unchecked; if in adolescence wealth has gratified every one of the increasing, though in essence natural, desires for excitement, for self-adornment, for self-advancement and self-prominence in every shape; if the Ego has been thus allowed to take the chief, almost the only, place in the woman's

common sense (*i.e.*, common mind), what is the inevitable result?

The common mind is stored with all that relates to self and takes up readily (in the balance) only those impressions and ideas which relate to self; and you have a completely *self-centred individual*, a mind isolated because it does not find in the world those with which it can, or cares to, communicate.

Though in no sense of the word an insane mind, its vision of everything (when the mind makes itself up) is distorted. It honestly does its best often to see, to be persuaded to other people's views, but, like a person with bad astigmatism, it cannot with the best will in the world see straight lines where others see them.

To such an egoist comes suddenly a grave disappointment. That which it ardently desired is out of reach or is lost; the balance is disturbed. Not only the reasoning faculty, as in Neurasthenia, but the subconscious and unconscious portions of the mind are thrown into violent disorder; the weakened moral powers, the debilitated, insufficiently exercised intuitive powers of

THE FEMININE MIND 31

the mind give way and disorganization reigns through *every part* of the body.

And, pathetic as it is, you can often see in the midst of this mental and physical chaos the old pampered Ego fighting hard for first place.

Such is the genesis of Hysteria. The unbalancing of the feminine type of mind, of the mind that has as its physical basis not only the grey matter that envelops the hemispheres of the brain, with which acute active consciousness is associated, and which is concerned mainly in the weighing of cause and effect; but also the white matter beneath it, with which the instinctive and more spiritual mind is connected, disturbance of which, if great, may involve even the centres of the lower brain and bring under its deranged mental control many functions which, in ordinary life, are beyond will power and automatic in their action. I have seen a hysterical patient at will reduce in five minutes the action of her heart from 88 to 18 beats a minute; and another take a large bowl of bread and milk and, at my command, arrest the food at the end of the œsophagus and return it at a signal, un-

altered, into a basin; or, if I ordered it, allow the food to pass direct into the stomach and at a given signal reject it, altered by the acid secretion of the stomach. Under strict conditions precluding imposture I have seen the body temperature sent up as much as 7 degrees in the course of half an hour, whilst paralysis and wasting, phantom tumours and a close imitation of every known disease, are quite the commonplace phenomena in hysterical patients at every hospital. Through one and all of these manifestations the prevailing egoism of the patient is generally apparent, and this has led to the belief, now known to be erroneous, that wilful effort is always consciously at work. This is not so; the patient is always herself deceived, though she may consciously add to her symptoms in her craving for attention and sympathy.

The one instance to which space restricts me is that of a man whom I knew as a patient for nearly thirty years.

In business, and aged about thirty when I first met him, he had considerable artistic taste, was emotionally religious, had some literary pretensions, was always *en pose*,

and was fond of asking people what, from his appearance, they would judge him to be, delighted always if the reply was a doctor, an editor, or a clergyman. Vain and self-important, he was always having his character written and quoting the laudatory paragraphs. He would discuss himself and his symptoms for hours, with gusto. He had, in succession, partial blindness, complete deafness and functional paralysis of several kinds. If he were crossed in any way he would have violent hysterical convulsions with aimless violence; while he took business reverses (he failed more than once) with placidity. After one of his later reverses he travelled round the world *en prince*, leaving his family to work their way out of his financial troubles. He lectured, and even wrote books about his travels, and, to his delight, obtained later a small literary post. He then had thoughts of purchasing a D.D. or LL.D. of some moribund American university. His end was characteristic. In a hysterical seizure he drew a penknife across his neck (not the first time he had inflicted superficial wounds on himself), and, though the cut was insignificant, it sufficed

to open the external jugular vein and he died of an air embolus in consequence.

He interested me greatly because, being intelligent and observant, he could give me —and did it with great delight—a good description of his various mental states. He was never hypochondriacal, and never alarmed about insanity, although he was conscious that his mind was occasionally out of accord with those of others. That to him was proof of superiority. He kept an exact register of all his thoughts, feelings and motives, especially of those that led up to and accompanied an acute attack. They would have filled several volumes and showed the possession of remarkable intuition in estimating the characters of others and many traces of real genius. He was an only child of very emotionably religious people, who destined him for the ministry and encouraged him, when a youth, to compose hymns and write sermons, and this early exaltation of his Ego unbalanced an otherwise fair specimen of the feminine mind type.

Resumé.—Under the simple analogy of a balance we see the fundamental process

THE FEMININE MIND

concerned in *making up one's mind*, and how essential it must be for mental health and comfort that our common sense should be fed with the impressions and ideas gathered from as wide a range of experience as possible. If the mind be nourished—as a result of faulty upbringing or by the force of circumstances—by an undue proportion of ideas that have relation to the self and its gratification, or indeed by one set of ideas of any kind, it falls unconsciously more and more out of touch with the general mind of the day (the Zeitgeist) and becomes isolated and may be keenly conscious of such isolation from which it cannot, unaided, escape.

When in this condition if it be balked in any of its extravagant and selfish aims, or even if the most natural of its instincts be denied to it, the result in the wide feminine mind type will show itself in extensive and manifold derangements (Hysteria), while in the reasoning masculine type any novel and unbalanceable idea or impression will produce a " theory " on which reason will construct a superstructure of dreads and terrors (Neurasthenia).

And I purpose to show in the following

chapters that the line of treatment is to take possession of—to impose one's will upon—the isolated mind and by suggestion (which may operate through various agents) to lead it back to contact with the general mind of humanity. That efficiently done, the cure will complete itself.

CHAPTER IV

NEURASTHENIA

i.e., loss of balance in the masculine type of mind

(*Synonyms:—Hypochondriasis, Psychasthenia,* Nervous *Debility, Nervous Breakdown, Depression, etc.*)

I HAVE adopted on the *lucus a non lucendo* principle and with a sole view to clearness, the best known of the above question-begging designations, Neurasthenia; for, as we have seen, the disorder is not due to nervous weakness but to the strictly normal activity of the mind in efforts to restore the balance in which mental health and comfort consist.

For just as the body maintains its balance in health by the ordered co-operation of all its organs, and, health being lost, sets in action certain phenomena (known as the symptoms of functional disease) with the sole object of the restoration of its equilibrium (which tendency used to be called the

Vis Medicatrix Naturæ), so the mind in a like state of instability directs her activities to a like end, *i.e.*, a restoration of balance.

In the mind, as we have seen, the cause of disturbance must be some circumstance, represented by impressions or ideas, to which the mind is unaccustomed and which it cannot therefore readily balance. These are either *sensations* which generally take their rise in some one of the abdominal organs, such as the liver, stomach or sexual apparatus, which have but very indirect connection with the highest brain centres, or certain strange *ideas*, that have a bearing on one's welfare, and which, because of their novelty, cannot be connected with any of our usual trains of thought and assimilated, *i.e.*, balanced.

Predisposing Causes of Neurasthenia.—The books give to *heredity* a prominent position among these, but its influence, according to my own statistics of about 800 cases, is negligible in Neurasthenia. The mistake has, I think, arisen from the common confusion of this disorder with Hysteria, in which a hereditary predisposition to instability is a strongly-marked feature.

NEURASTHENIA

As regards *overwork*, I unhesitatingly affirm that the influence of genuine, wholesome, all-round work will be found, on critical examination, to be very slight; though it is the favourite cause assigned by the patient. The classes of work that are baneful, even in moderation, are those that keep the individual out of active communion with his fellow-man, or that actually deprive the brain of work; such are routine employments, and those that offer no sufficient prize as stimulus to individual thought and enterprise, and those which necessitate the long habitual use of one or a few only of the mental faculties. To be health-giving, work must be varied, must necessitate free intercourse with other minds, and must provide that carrot in front of the donkey which alone can make it progress with alacrity. To the deadening effect of unsuitable work, even more than to the want of physical exercise, breakdowns are due. Co-operation from the active interest it generates in the workers' minds seems to me to have great possibilities in the prevention of all varieties of nervous disorder. What about *worry*? Its effect depends much on the

situation and the personality. I have known cases in which it had a curative effect as a stimulant, a way in which some great disaster will often act—pulling a man together, deciding him to new and more vigorous effort. But in blind alley employments, and there are many such, worry may act as the final straw to the overburdened camel; but, as I have said, it is not possible to lay down any rule for everything depends on the kind of worry and the predisposition of the mind. *Whatever tends to produce isolation of mind* is the one great antecedent condition to Neurasthenia. As long as even the most unstable of minds keeps itself among the crowd and is " in and of the world " it is on safe ground and in the most favourable state to regain any foothold temporarily lost. In proportion as you fail in contact with general humanity you admit self to too large a share in the common sense (common mind), every day opening the door wider to the Ego till at last it becomes master therein; and when that is the case the most trivial of impressions and ideas, as long as they have any bearing on self, become magnified in im-

portance until more or less everything that takes place comes to be regarded as having direct reference to self. This is the *hermit mind*, and it is the mind of nearly all Neurasthenics and of all Hysterics. I have known a man of splendid physique and accustomed to command rendered so self-conscious by prolonged isolation as to experience acute feelings of self-abasement in passing chattering workmen who were, as he imagined, engaged in criticizing his appearance and motives. Every reader who has suffered at all from Neurasthenia will understand how such a state of matters can come about. Most of the men who pass as proud and distant are sufferers from some form of Neurasthenia. They feel their isolation keenly but have become so abnormally sensitive that they cannot face the only remedy, the health-giving plunge into the great sea of humanity. Yet this isolation, which has such painful consequences, is rarely the fault of the sufferer, for, exclusive of those in whom it is engendered by the nature of their employment, it is usually the outcome of close application to study and most men of letters

and science experience it to some degree. Their devotion to a special line of work leads them unconsciously into the backwaters of life, and thus we often observe that really great men are exceedingly shy and reserved simply because they are neurasthenic, while the lesser fry, who have as motto " Ad majorem Mei gloriam," and self-advertisement as their object, tend to Hysteria quite as often as to Neurasthenia when their minds are off balance as a result of isolation. Thus Neurasthenia has come to be viewed as the malady of superior intellect. " Spiritus altos frangit et generosos," said old Burton, and in truth its victims among the thoughtless and uneducated are by comparison very few.

Strain and Stress must be reckoned among the predisposing influences. Puberty and the climacteric are the great natural periods of strain, and, as we shall see, sexual Neurasthenia is one of the most common disorders of young and vigorous men, while the many mental disturbances attending puberty and the climacteric in women assume, according to the type of mind of

the sufferer, the form either of Neurasthenia or of Hysteria.

Thus nerve weakness and mind weakness are in their whole development course and termination the very opposites of what we see in the diseases that still, in borrowed Greek garb, pass under their names, for nervous weakness involves real prostration, as you see in the worst stages of such acute diseases as typhoid fever and pneumonia, while mental weakness—Psychasthenia in a literal sense—is the characteristic of advanced brain disease and of senility. The Neurasthenic, using the term in our sense as indicative of mental instability, will indeed volubly assure you that he cannot stand upright; that he falls down after walking a few steps; that he cannot concentrate his mind on work; that the labour even of dressing himself is a formidable one; that he cannot recollect sometimes the most familiar names; in short, that his mind is going if not actually gone; but if you measure his total output of energy you will always find it *in excess of the average*, but extravagantly used, misdirected and dissipated in irrelevancies of thought and

action, tangled and confused to such a degree that endless patience and full knowledge of the individual and of his environment, and above all tact, are essential to the adviser who would undertake the responsibility of his direction. Is not the sufferer also perverse? Yes, and adverse to such a degree that a learned German has recently issued a pamphlet on Neurasthenia and kindred mental states, entitled *Zur theorie des Schizophrenen Negativismus.* Schizophrenic Negativism! What a name for the negative attitude which, by the way, is, under the circumstances, the only logical one in Neurasthenia as seen from the patient's standpoint. Resting, as we are all bound to do in unusual experiences, on the best theory he could find, he has logically built thereon a superstructure of disease, has generated by this mental bias many symptoms which tend to confirm him in the truth of his original theory, and, running in such grooves, he is suddenly countered by the blunt statement that he is altogether wrong by a doctor who thinks to carry the aforesaid strong position by a direct frontal attack. Try such strategy on the one-idea

man (the faddist) or on the doctrinaire socialist who dreams of a stable social balance, not knowing that in individual mind as in nations the very oscillations of the balance are life itself, and you will find plenty of Negativismus. No; if you are to prevail with the settled Neurasthenic you cannot expect often to succeed by a *coup de main* but must be content with some slower process, such as that of " running a parallel," after having first carefully mastered the processes that have led to his present state, and appraised the strength and disposition of the forces in opposition to you.

Let me give an instance of the use of such a parallel. A man, about thirty, a noted athlete, in perfect physical condition, in low, solemn tones complained of Syphilis. His conscience was clear but he had a pimple on his leg which he pointed to as the seat of infection. His physical strength was his great asset and his mind always directed to its maintenance. Having had to undergo medical examination in view of some appointment, the examiner had remarked that the pimple looked like the initial characteristic papule of Syphilis. Mercurial treat-

ment was started, and, aided by self-suggestion and vigorous skin friction with blue ointment, an eczematous state of the skin soon ensued. This, with other trivial symptoms, confirmed the patient in his fears. It was impossible to shake them. I then wrote on a piece of paper that I proposed to deceive him, placed it in a sealed envelope and gave it to a friend of the patient who accompanied him, telling him to keep it and return it to me unopened when I demanded it. I then said to the patient: " A clear case of rag-picker's disease (anthrax), infection probably arising from contamination of your clothing in some country laundry; if you read up the disease you will see that I am right. You will get quite well." In the absence of the mercurial frictions the eczema disappeared promptly, but a vigorous cough (a minor symptom of rag-picker's disease) developed. In a month, when the idea of Syphilis aroused only indignation in the patient's mind, I asked his friend to hand me the sealed letter. The patient read it and was delighted. He remained well and readily forgave the innocent deception. Was I not justified by my

Hippocratic graduation oath, a paragraph of which runs thus: "Et quoad potero, omnia ad ægrotorum corporis salutem conducentia cum fide procuraturum"?

It is a characteristic of Neurasthenia that the victims are generally in excellent physical health. Organic disease is rare even in inveterate cases, and when present has no part in the production of the mental complaint; a statement strictly true and easily explained, for although the patient is keenly concerned about his health, this concern is concentrated only on such disturbances of it *as he cannot account for*, and in these only can his mind reach no condition of equilibrium. Those which are visible, tangible and comprehensible, such as the organic diseases, not only does he meet with ordinary courage but often with indifference. Indeed, with the advent of organic disease Neurasthenia and Hysteria take their temporary departure, and so generally recognized is this that I have several times been asked by patients to inoculate them with the microbe of some definite disease because they preferred known dangers to the ghosts and shadows of disease that

haunted their minds. Influenza is often cited as an example to the contrary, but that disease is itself often vague in its symptoms and thus might legitimately come under the heading of novel impressions that are recognized causes of Neurasthenia; but, as a fact, the muscular and nervous debility that accompany and follow Influenza can but rarely be justly styled a real Neurasthenia with its attendant bogies and multiform complications.

There is no more common disorder than Neurasthenia, but it occurs so frequently in mild and transient forms, and seems to the victim so unreal and so inexplicable, that he hesitates to consult his friends, or even the doctors, and its existence is known only to himself, for, strange as it may seem, the Neurasthenic, later to haunt to his detriment many consulting-rooms, at first puts little faith in physic. There may be several reasons for this. I speak with the experience of a sufferer from this malady from thirteen to forty-one years of age, and of one who up to twenty-six years of age spent very considerable sums in fees, seeking relief therefrom and with very unsatisfactory

results. I longed to explain and to be understood, but was barely listened to. The diagnoses varied widely, from imagination, whatever that might mean, and liver disturbance, to incipient insanity, and the treatment was uniformly one with tonics, such as Strychnine, Quinine and Phosphorus, all of which aggravated my symptoms. One only—and he a homœopath—gave me a white crystalline powder, evidently, from what I now know, a bromide, which did relieve remarkably, but he demanded such an extravagant sum for the prescription that it was beyond my power to purchase it. In the midst of my worst attacks I was always in excellent general health and capable of walking thirty miles a day. It left me finally when I had the misfortune to be infected by a hospital patient, on my right index finger, with a severe and very chronic disease, and I can truly say that the exchange of diseases was a pleasant experience.

Many of the mild cases get well spontaneously, and even many of the severe ones pass off quickly under the restorative effect of the hard work that is required of most men in this world. Some find the power to

endure it till it vanishes by some change in their life or by some sudden adversity—for adversity however great is tangible and therefore steadies the mind. Courage and fortitude are of enormous assistance in recovery.

One charming old lady, for forty years the re-elected head of a religious community, gave me an account of the exceptionally severe and prolonged sufferings she had formerly endured. When I inquired as to treatment she replied simply that being the Will of God she had bowed to it and gone ahead at her work. She had found the philosopher's stone.

So important is it for the patient to remember that in work, even severe work, lies the best road to recovery, in all but a very few cases, that I need offer no apology for quoting one more individual experience.

In 188— I had a severe attack; the feeling of isolation from the rest of humanity, the sense of " unreality " in surrounding objects being most keen. The fear that I should suddenly lose self-control was ever with me, my special bogy being a fear lest I should be forced against my will to commit suicide

NEURASTHENIA

or some crime of violence. (To this obsession of suicide is, I find, traceable the popularity achieved by the safety razor.) Like most sufferers I slept and ate well. An eminent neurologist advised a walking tour down the Loire. I went, and for the three weeks it lasted suffered untold agonies, often begging the friend who accompanied me to place me safe in an asylum. I returned to London looking ill and worried, and was told by the same consultant to take at least six months' rest, and on no account to return to practice. My assistant, when informed of this, replied that I could take that holiday only when I had seen a number of people waiting to consult me. The next ten days were days of almost ceaseless night and day work, but I was absolutely well ere they passed and remained perfectly free from any return for several years.

Nothing is more frequently seen in the daily papers than the statement that severe depression had preceded an attempt at suicide, and the idea has become quite general that neurasthenic states (nervous breakdowns) may lead to a tragedy. Nothing is further from the truth. Melan-

cholia, an insane state marked by *delusions*, silence, and general mental torpor, is of course a frequent precursor of suicide, but Melancholia is the very opposite of Neurasthenia, and of anything that can legitimately come under the latter designation. To clear this point, in which I was myself secretly interested, I made it a duty to interview several people who had made determined, but fortunately ineffectual, efforts at self-destruction. Strange to say all were, after recovery, willing to explain their state antecedent to the attempt. There were five such cases and in not one had there been any prior fear of the act nor any neurasthenic condition of mental suffering. Two said that they were dazed and oppressed, and neither thought nor cared about the consequence of their act; the other three that the act seemed at the time quite the most natural thing to do. I have never known of a case in which Neurasthenia or any allied condition led to self-destruction. The fear of it in the Neurasthenic is indeed keen but is the dread of a dread, though when, as sometimes happens, some drug habit has been contracted by the sufferer

he may deliberately destroy himself. This however is due to an unwise attempt to suddenly and completely break the bonds of drug slavery, and the consequent unendurable suffering, or to despair at his failure. In Hysteria, as we shall see later on, the drama of suicide is often enacted as a comedy but may be overdone and end in tragedy.

The Bogy (or Obsession) in Neurasthenia.—The most outstanding feature in Neurasthenia is the *bogy* (the phobia of the text-books). Given an intimate knowledge of the patient's modes of thought and general life, his *bogy may be foretold* with accuracy. Nothing impresses a sufferer more than this proof of the doctor's foreknowledge. It is arrived at very simply, for it represents, of course, that which is most abhorrent to the particular patient, being in its essence only a supreme dread. The bogy represents the theory (the counter-weight adopted for purposes of mental balance) formed to account for novel impressions and ideas of which the causation is not apparent to the mind, or some logical deduction from that theory, and it always relates to self. Injury

to mind or body, to self-love or reputation is the basis. *The Bogy of insanity* has its source in forms of mental discomfort such as the dream-like or fog-like sensation, or the feeling of isolation, or the apparently threatened loss of self-control and consequent involuntary suicide or crime. One form of *train fear* and *ship fear* is based on this. *The Bogy of sudden and violent death* is connected with *fear of open or of confined spaces, of water and of fire*. *The Bogy of disease* is not quite of the same class. Suffering or disfiguration, and the risk of becoming abhorrent to humanity, are dreaded, but any fear of death in the ordinary way is rarely acknowledged by Neurasthenics, and, whatever be the disease to which they eventually succumb, it must be acknowledged that they meet death with calmness, failing to realize that it can be unaccompanied by the horrors which in imagination they have attached to it. One of the worst cases I ever attended—a man who for years varied his bogy almost every week though all had the fear of some disease as foundation—when dying of dropsy due to heart disease of old standing, loudly

intermitted the remark, "That is d——nonsense," when the clergyman referred to him in prayer by his bedside as "our dying brother." *The Bogy of injury to self-esteem* is at the bottom of that jealousy which haunts some Neurasthenics even while they carefully explain the baselessness of the obsession which they cannot shake off. *The Bogy of loss of good repute* is often put in some one of the following ways: "Suppose I were to enter a railway carriage and an old man were to get in at the last moment and I were to lose self-control and attack him. Imagine my disgrace as a commercial traveller known all down the line." Or, "Suppose a clerk in my office happened to be in the Strand at a moment that I turned round and that he thought I was looking at a loose woman. Imagine the ridicule at my place of business." Or, "Suppose I, in a sudden loss of self-control, put poison into a water-bottle in a public waiting-room, and that it killed someone, and that my act had been observed. Imagine my situation as a prominent member of the Bar." Far-fetched and absurd as such fears may seem to the

sound and healthy they are quite ordinary forms of self-torment to men of intellect and who are perfectly and absolutely sane but Neurasthenic.

A large volume might be written solely on the hues assumed by different bogies. They are as various as the occupations and minds of the sufferers, but never are they in any sense of the word *delusions* but always and only *fears founded on theory*. There is a special prominence given to the numbers 3 and 7 by many neurasthenic minds and which is difficult adequately to account for, but the origin of the idea is probably theological and based on the Trinity, the seven mortal sins, and the seven cardinal virtues.

And here, for the relief of any Neurasthenic reader, I may answer a question often put to me in great anxiety: " But what *would* happen to me if I actually lost my self-control? " The answer is, an *hysterical paroxysm*. The feminine mind, never acutely concerned about consequences, makes no effort, in the condition of strain felt so acutely by neurasthenic masculine minds, to inhibit or restrain itself, but simply

NEURASTHENIA 57

lets itself go and explodes in tears, shrieks or muscular contortions before the stress becomes unendurable, while the masculine mind in Neurasthenia, dreading possible disaster, or at least ridicule, keeps a firm hand on its strange impulses and suffers acutely in consequence. The feeling is like that experienced in a trotting race when you require all your muscular power to keep the horse from breaking into a gallop and fear every moment that he will overpower you.

I have more than once seen this state of tension end in hysterical sobbings and convulsions in emotional Neurasthenics, and have remarked that it brought quick relief; but one cannot recommend it in treatment since self-control is a rare enough virtue and one to be encouraged most of all in the victims of such mental disequilibration as we are discussing.

But the reader must not conclude that all cases of Neurasthenia or of Hysteria are typical like those I have selected for illustration. In minds more or less compounded in varying proportions of the masculine and feminine types of mind Neurasthenia and Hysteria may touch or

even overlap at certain points, but no two disorders in pure mind types are in their leading characters more distinct.

A clear and intimate knowledge of the underlying causations and the many ramifications of Neurasthenia is essential to the man who would treat the disease with success, and only the doctor who has himself suffered can fully understand the language of the patient and appreciate the sufferings that attend this, the most painful, and, in its origin, the least understood of disorders.

CHAPTER V

THE TREATMENT, ETC., OF NEURASTHENIA

THE following are the essential points:

First and foremost, no time or pains must be spared in obtaining a clear mental picture of the patient, avoiding of course all irrelevant details. A good plan is to shut the eyes and to let the patient talk, even if he consumes an hour or two in the process. *Nothing is unimportant.* Apparently trivial matters often furnish useful guides. You thus obtain a map of the disorder, and view its source, and all that has contributed to its development. You further note the points on which your attack may be directed.

It is a mistake to stop the patient; let him unburden himself and give, unchecked, his opinions. By so doing you learn his motives and his reasons and note the way in which his mind naturally works, and as you

will have to work with him, it is essential to obtain this knowledge so that your treatment may commend itself to his judgment. We must have no more Negativismus than we can help.

Secondly, having pumped him quite dry, a most careful physical examination must be made and full notes thereof taken; nothing should be left out lest the omitted part assume later on to the anxious patient's mind the probable place of origin of his malady. Often in past days has the patient said, " You have taken no blood for analysis," adding significantly, " I think you will find the disease there." Therefore, however apparent be the underlying cause of his complaint to yourself, you cannot afford to skip any part of the examination.

I always take my own specimens and submit them to well-known skilled analysts, and ask the patient to post them, allowing the report to be sent direct to him if any preference for that course be shown. Neurasthenics, without meaning any offence, are often very suspicious.

In three or four days, when the reports

have come in and been considered, I ask the patient to call and hand him my *written opinion*.

This written opinion—with the reasons on which each conclusion is based—is the keynote of treatment. It shows the patient that you are sure of yourself, and in the present day, with our many aids to diagnosis, a careful man is fully justified in self-confidence. This document is a great stay to the patient in the moments that are sure to come when old doubts will reappear. I have had proof of its efficacy in the many cases in which the decided tone of the opinion has alone kept the patient to the line of safety when verbal advice had faded. One lady indeed thus reproached me: "Why didn't you write that letter at first instead of saying, 'In my opinion you will get well.'" Even long after they have recovered patients will keep such a letter and feel a security against relapse in its occasional reperusal.

Thirdly, deal with the Bogy. To foretell the bogy to the patient is to rob it of much of its importance and appearance of solidity. But though you may thus sap

its credit you must not at once proceed to a direct attack on its person. On the contrary, sometimes you must run a counter-attraction, a rival; sometimes you may pull the bogy to pieces bit by bit, or again you may dig the ground from under it. Charge it in the open, as hypnotists so often do, and you will come off a very bad second, and you cannot afford any reverse. Many cases of Neurasthenia are of a very chronic type and in them the bogy may be too firmly "set" to yield to any of the aforesaid measures. In these I find great help from an "*Infallible.*" Now an Infallible is a medicine that cures without being taken, a formula of great mental potency, but composed of real drugs capable of actually and really displacing the enemy, but which it would be unadvisable for the patient to take regularly. Therefore the prescription is marked "Emergency only," and is carefully guarded by the verbal direction: "Take a dose of this only if you feel that you have come to your last ditch." Now the typical Neurasthenic, being an anxious man, says to himself in an emergency: "I will not take this medicine lest it should

injure me. The doctor told me that, though certain in effect, it was a little risky by reason of its potency." Or again: "If I take a dose and it fail my last hope will be gone, I will reserve it for a still worse attack;" and one peculiarity of all crises in which the bogy plays the principal part is that they cease just before they become absolutely insupportable. The following will illustrate this point. A friend and patient agreed to undertake, by my strong advice, a voyage to Japan, but though in excellent physical health—despite a stay for months in various northern nursing homes which had converted a passing Neurasthenia, to which he was subject, into a confirmed state of auto-suggestion with threatening paralysis as the bogy—he was most nervous about leaving London. He was given an Infallible with the usual directions, and on returning to England he placed the bottle, still sealed, on my mantelpiece with the remark: "That medicine cured me though I never drew the cork."

Fourthly, work must be insisted on. A man's usual occupation, if it be at all congenial to him, and if it provide abundant

means of meeting and conversing with his fellows, is the best. It should be of a kind that, once started, means *compulsory* regularity and attention. All other measures will fail until you have secured this essential to success. In nine cases out of ten it is the *only* treatment necessary. Of course you will find it hard to persuade the patient to this salutary course. He will object, " You make me well and I will return to work," putting the cart before the horse; or, " I shall die if I work," but " I will work if I die," is the view that you must insist on. The benefit of work is so obvious that one is puzzled to account for the "rest cure" fad unless it arise from a refusal of battle for the sake of the adviser's peace and quiet. Eminent writers from the dawn of literature, most of them sufferers, are absolutely unanimous on the benefit of work in all neurasthenic states. " In idleness alone is there perpetual despair," said Carlyle. Galen called idleness " Maximum animi nocumentum." " This body of ours, when it is idle and knows not how to bestow itself, macerates and vexes itself with cares, griefs, false fears, discontents and suspicions, and

is never at rest," adds Burton, and one might continue similar quotations *ad infinitum*.

You may very occasionally meet a Neurasthenic who may need rest for some good reason, and rest will usually fatten, but for the vast majority whose minds are only disorientated, and who are free from any organic disease that could benefit by such measures, rest is absolutely the one thing to be avoided, the one condition, especially if combined with isolation, that may be relied on to seriously aggravate their state. For those whose only occupation in life is the so-called pursuit of pleasure, who ignore that pleasure depends little on externals, and is in any case restricted to narrow limits of capacity in man, and that games, hobbies and foreign travel are but poor substitutes for regular work, for such the outlook in Neurasthenia is a serious one.

Truisms indeed, but how often forgotten!

Fifthly, seek out the ambition latent in all of us. The patient at his first interview will give the clue, and it is for the doctor to make of it a lever. But " a stout heart for a stiff brae," and the patient must creep

to the goal of his special desire if he cannot run; he must at once get a move on in any case. Most of us know by experience how small the prize when it is won, but we all remember how useful was the spur of hope that kept us to the way. More neglected truisms!

Sixthly. Under this heading we may place all other agents. Of these *Hypnotism* is but suggestion "writ large," and on suggestion in some form reliance must be placed throughout all the treatment of Neurasthenia. In my experience it is rarely wise or even useful to place the patient under full hypnotic influence; suggestions implanted in the trance state never long survive the awakening, for their impression is not on the conscious mind. They are like branches carelessly tied, not grafted, to a tree trunk and they early wither. Marvellous results were ascribed to Hypnotism by Dr Charcot in the old days at La Salpêtrière, but the disease was Hysteria, and the innate tendency of the Hysteric to take a leading part in any function was forgotten, and, as recognized later on when the patients overdid the game, the doctors were either the victims

NEURASTHENIA

of deception, or failed, as I think, to fully interpret the phenomena.

Food as an agent may be of great utility, especially where the original disturbing impressions are located in some one of the digestive organs. In them the results of a reduced dietary are most gratifying. My rule, in such cases, is to reduce nourishment to the point at which the weight, if a fairly normal one, can just be maintained. If the patient be obese, weight should be taken off by a graduated dietary, plus exercises; the latter never to be omitted from the plan. For the Neurasthenic in good physical condition, and over thirty years of age, two meals a day—a good breakfast and a good late dinner—usually suffice. For the first fortnight a few sandwiches or biscuits and a cup of black coffee may be allowed at midday. If there be present active dyspeptic symptoms, half a pint of very hot and weak China tea (boiling water poured on a closed infusing-spoon till a pale shade of the fluid is produced, when the spoon is withdrawn) with a slice of lemon may advantageously be ordered at 11 a.m. and 5 p.m. It is as efficient as, and much more agreeable than,

the plain hot water usually advised. Maté may be substituted for the China tea. Indian teas, unless very fine, are not good, and milk and sugar as additions are anathema to all real tea-lovers.

Yet, since you should never oppose a Neurasthenic if you can honestly meet him, and as many are shocked at the idea of but two simple meals a day, so often have they been assured of the benefits of "feeding up," you must now and then have recourse to a diet fad, and when you have to reduce the amount of food Vegetarianism is the best system to select. There is no food system that can be good—or even safe—for every one and everywhere, and I do not promiscuously advise Vegetarianism, but in suitable cases I must confess that I have seen great and durable benefit from its adoption, not only in nervous disorders but in gout, dyspepsia, rheumatism and many other diseases. Its effect, when beneficial, is chiefly due in my opinion to simple all-round reduction in the amount of food assimilated, for chemical analysis abundantly proves that, until the digestive organs can accommodate themselves to the altered

NEURASTHENIA 69

circumstances, much of the vegetable material eaten (satisfactory as seems the chemistry of its elements on paper) is thrown off by the bowel. Incidentally this makes for regularity of evacuation. Like all other reduced food systems it tends to lessen the desire for alcohol and the craving for tobacco, and a few glasses of good light wine and half a dozen cigarettes a day should be the limit in Neurasthenia. No novel food system, least of all the ones that restrict their votaries to fruits or to meat, should ever be undertaken unless some instructed and responsible person be taken as judge of its effects, for all abstinence and fasting so clear the mind, and the result is so cheering and delightful, that actual damage to bodily health may easily ensue ere the patient be aware of his danger. Tuberculosis is a special risk in this connection. Persons who speak of *drugs* as if they belonged to some special order in nature, marked off by definite lines from foods, are misinformed. No such water-tight compartments are known to chemistry; neither is there any standard of health by relation to which substances can be classed as good

or bad. That only is beneficial which adequately supplies a need in the particular person. Even such things as common salt, oxygen or ozone, are deadly poisons when used in excess. Thus drugs whose full action is known have their use in certain eventualities, if not employed merely to mask a symptom at the expense of possible subsequent mischief.

Mental exercises are during the course of an attack very useful, but they should, as *formal exercises*, be stopped directly the patient has got over his attack, for our minds are so constituted that strict affirmations readily call up a negative picture. I welcome the recent rise in London of a school of mental exercise and mind culture, for the benefits to be expected of wise schooling in concentration and regulation of thought are of incalculable value to the community in general, and to business and professional men in particular; even the general physical health may be improved thereby.

The mental exercises of use in Neurasthenia are of a very simple order and should consist in a series of practical resolutions, said out loud, with the mind concentrated

on the thoughts, each morning when at rest. Thus, "I will get up at 8 a.m., I will breakfast at 9," and so on with the simple duties of the day, and a quarter of an hour should be devoted, in quietude, each evening to a review of the result attained. Space prevents me from giving more than an outline of a system that, simple as it is, if faithfully carried out, is productive of much good. Life is thereby regularized and habit soon makes such regularity easy and natural.

Finally, there is one most important point. It is always foolish for anyone to make health a subject of concern, for discussions about disease may by suggestion produce actual disorder. In Neurasthenia it is specially pernicious, and the patient must be put on his honour not to consult doctors, to read medical books, suggestive advertisements, or even articles on health in the press, and he must learn to check, and expel resolutely from his mind, any doubts, or even any thoughts, about his own health. The physician must lend his aid in the same direction, and, unless under special circumstances, should not see the patient after his

written opinion with full directions has been given for at least six weeks or longer, and then only on condition that the simple measures advised shall have all been fairly observed. Any difficulty that may arise in the interval is best dealt with by letter. The one aim of all treatment should be to make the patient independent of the doctor, and no cure is worthy the name that does not secure this end.

Sexual Neurasthenia.—The matter is so important, and in some of its aspects so misunderstood, and moreover sexual Neurasthenia itself gives such a perfect example of the origin and growth of all Neurasthenic states, that I need little excuse for making brief reference to the subject.

We all know that boys at the impressionable age at which they attend school are apt to be mentally contaminated by evil companionship; the boy himself being unaware of the consequences that will ensue later on when he wakes to the full consciousness of life—at from twenty to twenty-six years of age. At that age, under the strain of indoor work and of the natural perturbations that attend on the development of a

function in its meaning more racial than individual, he becomes listless and self-centred, and in that state may incidentally drop across some quack advertisement or some specious book that, under the benign guise of giving advice to young men, hides the most damnable attempts on his health and purse. Insanity, brain softening, consumption, fits, and especially a failure or *loss of virility* are, according to the writers, but a few of the dire consequences of certain bad habits. All lies! for the habits referred to, objectionable as they are, have no power to produce any of these consequences, and beyond abasing the youth unduly in his own estimation, and at the worst producing a transient and easily-curable local hypersensitiveness and some functional disturbance of the sympathetic nervous system, do no harm whatever.

But sexual Neurasthenia has been started, and though any experienced doctor could readily prove to the sufferer that neither physical disease nor insanity are even possible consequences of his acts, yet the impeachment of his virility makes a bogy hard to overcome. Any practical test is

out of the question, and if tried would, by reason of the nervous doubts implanted, probably fail, and thus confirm the prognosis of the quack and establish the bogy more firmly in his seat. Nor is it easy to reassure the patient, even when his local symptoms have been cured, to his entire satisfaction. Rigid censorship must, of course, be established over evil thoughts, a regime which, hard at first, is found, if persevered in, to be attainable; while everything that may prove suggestive must be taboo. These measures may re-establish the sufferer in his own estimation, but the question of loss of virility will often remain behind to rankle in the breast, and break out anew into a blaze of fear if and when marriage is contemplated. The mind of the sufferer, long the seat of sensuality, takes quite an erroneous view of the aims and duties of matrimony, and, being unable to realize the picture of a pure and simple love, free of even the knowledge or thought of evil, still less of desire, pictures the future bride as a sensual ogress to be appeased. In many cases the neurasthenic man, knowing little of woman's instinctive nature, has not even the wisdom

NEURASTHENIA

to keep his fears to himself, and the wife becomes distressed by her husband's nervousness, the foundation of which she cannot fathom. Fortunately, in the worst cases, those that do not get well of themselves, a doctor, by his knowledge of the innate negativism of Neurasthenia, and by application thereof in merely forbidding any attempt for a month and by taking the wife into his confidence, can secure a satisfactory result. In justice I should add that the foregoing condition of matters may arise in any neurotic man and without any antecedent evil practices at all.

If the doctor knows of the bogy in advance he may forestall its evil machinations as the following case will show.

A gentleman in perfect physical health but in a very neurasthenic state consulted me. It was many years ago and I had not learnt then what I now know. He suggested for six weeks prior to his marriage a daily subcutaneous injection of strychnine as a tonic, and I fell in with his views. All seemed to go well till a few hours before the ceremony, when he came to me in a state of such extreme nervousness that I feared he

would never face the marriage at all. At my wits' end I said, "Well, in any case you had better have the last injection." He consented, with supreme indifference and in profound gloom. My last tabloid of strychnine was gone, and, doubting the wisdom of informing him of the fact lest thereby I should increase his fears, I dissolved a tabloid of $\frac{1}{20}$th grain of morphia and injected it. The dose was, I knew, too small to do any harm, but I had no foreknowledge of the actual result. He came in boisterously to see me some weeks later and remarked, "I don't know what you gave me but I would have married forty women that morning if necessary."

Then it dawned on me that a sedative was what he had all along wanted; not an excitant such as strychnine. The morphia simply allayed all doubts, and, as he was quite unaccustomed to the drug, the effect lasted for two or three days.

Such is sexual Neurasthenia, the most typical and amenable to cure of all the varieties if once it be treated reasonably, but it must be remembered that every local functional disorder must be always put to

NEURASTHENIA

rights before the mental state will yield to any treatment.

General Considerations in the Treatment of all Cases of Neurasthenia.—Complete sympathy and understanding between doctor and patient must exist in any successful treatment of Neurasthenia. In fact, the doctor must be the confidant and trusted friend of the sufferer, and, by his accurate memory of details and his readiness to respond by letter to any query, prove that he is keeping the patient and his difficulties ever before his mind's eye. A mental state in the patient must be met by the exercise of mental faculties on the side of the adviser. Frequent interviews, as I have elsewhere said, are never advisable, and as a practical physician I have often recognized the evil effect, in all sickness, of unnecessary visits and their bad influence in leading a doctor, at the call of some insistent but unimportant symptom, to depart from that strict line of treatment which a first careful examination of the patient has determined as the path towards cure. In Neurasthenia the patient is abnormally observant and critical in his study of the

physician's character and knowledge, and brusqueness, so often adopted as the cloak of ignorance, will raise opposition, ridicule and contempt in the patient's mind; while the "Cheer up, old fellow" attitude must be justly condemned as foolish. In Neurasthenia it is definitely the first step that counts, and if it be a false one the patient may be landed on the slope of a terrible descent. We have all met chronic and now hopeless cases of this disease in which honest but faulty methods adopted in the early treatment have been responsible for the final disaster. I could name several now living who still hug the bogy of a paralysis that has never materialized, and who, like the nervous lady looking under the bed for the burglar, daily search for signs of its coming, and, incredible as it may sound, one of them was urged to give up a prosperous, active life and devote himself to "a garden in the suburbs," because one day, for some unaccountable reason, he felt a dread in passing a certain house; another, a prosperous dentist, because several times he had felt anxious about his breathing if more than three people

NEURASTHENIA

were together in a room; while a third, formerly an active city merchant, was condemned because he developed, by way of bogy, an unreasonable fear of bankruptcy and the workhouse; all specimens, as every Neurasthenic knows, of the most ordinary obsessions, which would have passed away in the active work of life, but were now rooted and nourished by constant self-analysis in the only occupation, "complete rest," advised by some indifferent or thoughtless doctor who suggested insanity as the probable consequence of perseverance in work. Now that it is too late these people are miserably sane, occupied only with self-study and the discussion of fancied grievances; for let us remember that to the active mind rest is impossible, and that, in default of larger interests with which to concern itself, it will turn over and over—magnifying in the process — the most trivial concerns of a small household. Even the comparative mercies of insanity, with the oblivion of its fixed but false balance, is denied to these poor sufferers.

I admit, of course, that there are rare instances in which, for very special reasons,

rest may legitimately be advised in the early stages of Neurasthenia, and I know that certain organic brain diseases, in their beginnings, may present symptoms that can sometimes be mistaken for functional mental disorder, *i.e.*, for a mere loss of balance. As a young man I made such mistakes myself and have seen others make them, but the early symptoms of such organic diseases as general paralysis of the insane and disseminated cerebro-spinal sclerosis, very, very, rarely take the form of Neurasthenia, for the loss of balance which they simulate is that which is characteristic of the wider disturbance seen in the disordered feminine mind, namely, Hysteria.

CHAPTER VI

HYSTERIA

i.e., loss of balance in the feminine type of mind

PART I.—A STUDY OF THE FEMININE TYPE OF MIND

IF Neurasthenia be an inappropriate word to denote disequilibration in the masculine type of mind, what shall we say of Hysteria as adapted to the same phenomenon in the feminine one, for its very derivation denotes womb disorder pure and simple, though men of the Latin race are frequently the sufferers from an advanced form of it, and it is by no means uncommon, though usually in a milder variety, among males in the United States and in Great Britain. But we have practically no choice of names for the vast symptom-complex with which we have to deal is known all the world over only as Hysteria.

I gave in my third chapter a brief sketch of the feminine type of mind. Volumes would be required to do full justice to it, and behind these volumes would have to

be a mind of wide comprehension and great impartiality, stored with a varied experience of the most intimate sides of humanity. Therefore, if my description falls short, I fail in large company and because of my necessary limitations.

That mind is in a sense represented in the brain there can be no doubt. How it is represented, what is the relationship between the two, no one can say, though there is scarcely a philosopher that has not considered himself within touch of the answer, and the physiologist of my younger days felt sure that he possessed a simple and complete one. A clearer day has dawned and the modern man of science confesses that he can but state, to quote almost his identical words, that in some way mind makes matter, and that, from what to us is the void, a function calls for an organ and the necessary organ, adapted to the desirable function, is made: that physiology makes anatomy and not *vice versa*. It is the old " Fiat Lux " coming into its own again.

But these altitudes concern us little; what we have to understand is that accord-

HYSTERIA

ing to accurate observations certain portions of the brain act as transmitters of certain functions of the mind, that in general the cortex or upper segment of the cerebral hemispheres acts thus with regard to the reasoning faculties and the lower segment with what is called the subconscious or subliminal mind; not that we need attach any special value in this connection to the word reason, nor underrate the subconscious position of the mind because its *pied-à-terre* is the lower brain segment, for it is the seat of the emotions, of the wonderful and incomprehensible instincts and of genius.

The feminine type of mind occupies a much greater area of the brain than does the masculine, and presumably that is the explanation of its wider range, its greater capacity and its relative incomprehensibility; but it has the defects of its qualities, and in that lies its weakness. More rarely do we find a perfect feminine type, and far more often, because its complexity implies greater tendency to instability, do we find complete freedom from some disturbance; for it is a rule throughout nature that the

greater the complexity the greater the instability, the tendency on slightly adverse conditions to larger disturbance, and thus it happens that the feminine type of mind, though higher in facility and more extensive in its powers than the masculine, is but rarely seen in perfection; that imperfect types are the rule, and the imperfections more glaring to view and more numerous and more disastrous in effect than such as follow on imperfect forms of the masculine type. It is easy to sum up all the possible disabilities and failures of the latter; those of the former are as numerous as are its varieties of normal function. No region of the body, and not one of its functions, is safe from perversion when the feminine mind loses its hold over balance; not even what are known as the automatic and reflex powers are safe from interference. Permutations and combinations, to use a mathematical term, are then the rule of the day.

I do not propose to treat you to a compendium of the many strange efforts that have been made to define Hysteria, some of them extravagant and all conflicting. What is to be said of the unconscious

humorist who, defining woman as an "organism revolving around a womb," proceeds gravely to show how the orbit may be disturbed by pathological uterine states; or of his colleagues who assert that the functions of the womb are "strictly mechanical," and that it is certain outlying nerve centres that are answerable, by radiation, for all evil consequences; or of the grave physician who thinks he has really solved the whole problem when he calls Hysteria "an explosion," but deigns to add, out of charity for weaklings or possibly scoffers, "Nature having no outlet for superfluous energies, the whole system becomes disordered"; or again, of the Viennese professor who finds the solution in the "sundering of consciousness," as if ideas were tied like faggots into bundles; or of the American professor who sagely remarks, "Hysteria is essentially a psychosis as distinguished from Neurasthenia, which is a neurosis," precisely, just as the world is not a spinning globe but a globe that is spinning. In one matter they all agree, namely, in an equal anxiety about the pathology. Now pathology is a resultant,

a physical change, not the process that instigated it. It is as if the pilot, neglecting navigation and the law of storms, and refusing to apply his mind to anything but to defects, spent his time exclusively in examining his craft for signs of damage and refused to take any measures of precaution in times of danger till he had discovered them, and ascribed some crowning disaster solely to the started planks or the rusty bolts previously found, or, failing such, adopted the theory of an explosion.

One of the medical philosophers, however, puts his finger on a very sore place. When speaking of the so-called "neuromimesis" in Hysteria, he very pertinently asks: "How can memory set up a disease it has never seen? The disease (Hysteria) must be in psychic centres, but unconsciously; possibly a disease of œsthesodic cells of the cerebral hemispheres." The least critical of readers will rub his eyes. Memory of course is out of the question and must be dismissed, with costs against the writer, from the suit; as for disease being existent in a psychic centre, disease *a post hoc* existing as an *ante hoc* and in a psychic centre, *i.e.*, in an

HYSTERIA

abstraction! I give the quotation as a useful and very bad example of the false coin that finds currency in some circles. There is no real mystery at all, and the answer is extremely simple. Hysteria, being a loss of balance in the feminine type of mind, is a disorder of the *whole brain*, of the *whole mind*, and will therefore involve any or every function and throw any or every organ of the body upon the defensive; for functional disorder (the only kind in which Hysteria develops itself) is, as translated by its symptoms, but the natural effort made by any organ, for the sake of the maintenance of the general bodily equilibrium of health, to keep itself to the point of due co-operation with all other organs. That is why we may have any and every functional disorder in Hysteria. The difficulties of the medical casuists are easily solved if studied on the ordinary principles of science and if we free ourselves from the tyranny of theory-begging words. It brings to mind the nursery couplet—

> " O what a tangled web we weave
> When first we practise to deceive "—

but without, of course, ascribing to anyone voluntary deception. Real science concerns herself with simplification, not with complication, and in keeping to simple lines we shall save ourselves many a self-deception. Disorder and disturbance in any and every function of the body is what we then reasonably expect, and what we get, in every case of Hysteria, while as to the form and kind it will assume that will depend upon the individual patient's special bent of mind and upon surrounding circumstances: it may be blindness, deafness or muteness; loss of the power to move by will any one or more of the voluntary muscles and thus take the shape of a motor paralysis; or, leaving movement unimpaired, we may have the symptoms of a sensory paralysis, loss of the sense of touch, of temperature, of weight or of pain confined to a limb or a portion of a limb, or scattered promiscuously over the whole body; or we may have spasmodic contractions or absolute rigidities, discolorations or blanching of the skin, wasting due to local nutritional interferences, convulsions that may be quite partial, unilateral or general; or perversions of function may

be a prominent feature and the secretions of various organs may be altered in different ways; or, again, the will-power may extend its accustomed sway and obtain partial control over the usually automatic and reflex powers; or, strangest of all, psychic phenomena of a marvellous order may develop, in which the mind may seem to project itself, to partially disengage itself from its physical basis in the brain, as we see in certain spiritualistic performances, the best mediums for which are those that are endowed with a feminine type of mind, whatever their sex. That the absence of light is an essential to success in these demonstrations does not, in itself, prove them to be the result of imposture, conscious or unconscious, for it is possible that light may have some definite and intimate relationship to mind. While many of the demonstrations I have seen have been beyond my powers of explanation, I have witnessed none that I could assert were decisively superhuman or due to agencies other than of the human order, while the constant and irritating intermixture of most phenomena with imposture—pro-

bably not wilful in many cases—tends to confirm the candid observer in his views as to their dependence on subconscious human agency, for were it otherwise the question would arise: Why spoil a genuine and wonderful manifestation of psychic power by imposture unless you accept the theory that evil and lying infra-human spirits take a Puck-like part in the game, careless of the loss of credit involved in the adoption of such devices?

As a strictly impartial critic I can only regard spiritualistic manifestations as excellent examples of a feebly-developed feminine mind-type in a state of disorder, induced, as disorder in all of that type can easily be induced, by self-suggestion or by the suggestions of place, time and other minds. The audience, the dramatic setting and the suggestion are the three essentials in all hysterical as in all spiritualistic performances, and the reason of this is to be found in a special development of the Ego, the self, which, as we found when dealing with Neurasthenia, is also the chief factor in the long series of trouble in that complaint. Why should

HYSTERIA

the mental isolation form of this exaggeration of the self be productive of so much mischief? It is a practical matter and sufficiently important to demand our notice.

The Ego.—We know experimentally that in certain animal communities there is such a perfect unity of purpose as regards the well-being of the society and the perpetuation of the race that the life of the individual is if necessary sacrificed, without compunction, to those ends. We may take the bees and ants as examples of such perfect communes, and, as is well known, you cannot long keep an isolated individual, separated from his society, alive and well, however favourable be the environment you may arrange. When it is a question of gregarious animals living in moderate-sized flocks and with a more restricted community sense, such as the parrots, starlings and other flock-forming birds, you may indeed rear a single individual if captured while young, but failure often ensues, and in any case, if the captive be liberated after even a short confinement, he is not again received into the flock. Even in animals, then, a certain

development of what I call the "common mind" is seen under most conditions of life in common, and the animal that would live a happy normal life, or indeed any life at all, has to subordinate his Ego to the general mind of his community, which latter acts in some of the most material affairs of life, such, for instance, as migration in birds, and the formation of regular armies for attack, or even for a deliberate campaign, as in the ants, with one purpose as one mind. For this and other good reasons we may conclude that animals possess the same kind of mind, but of course much smaller in amount and more restricted in its range of ideas, as ourselves, and that therefore such of them as live habitually only in flocks and herds each possess a common mind (a share of the community mind), as well as a purely individual one. If isolation be then obviously in some way harmful to them we can readily understand that it will lead to far greater mischief in the human item of our modern communities, and indeed we actually witness among ourselves the same phenomena as in animals, namely the ex-

HYSTERIA

pulsion from society of individuals that do not conform to its general spirit, such as criminals, tramps, beggars and loafers, who are often free from intentional and deliberate desire to be bad and often possess many excellent individual qualities. These examples of this our human jetsam, as Lombroso and others who have closely studied them show, develop, after expulsion, a progressively anti-social spirit, becoming mentally more and more abnormal; though it is well to remark that in spite of their habits and unfavourable surroundings they do not in undue proportion become insane. Among the well-to-do and those fed and maintained by Christian charity an over-cultivation of the self leads to a similar perversion of the common mind (the latter then containing in its elements too large a proportion of the Ego), and, unless this is checked by the freest association in work and active competition, it necessarily becomes more and more perverted until the Ego occupies the whole mind when mental isolation is complete and severe forms of Hysteria develop. It is true the public rarely come across such individuals, for they are kept sedulously

from view by sensitive and kind friends and relations, and only doctors know from experience in what large numbers they exist.

In the active masculine type of mind, a type limited almost strictly to conscious functions, this isolation is also keenly felt, and forms, as we saw in a previous chapter, its chief distress, and just because it is so keenly appreciated the fear of insanity is the commonest of the theories (bogies) based thereupon; but in the feminine type, with its far wider basis of consciousness, instinct and other powers, its relation to a far larger area of brain, consciousness plays a much less conspicuous part, and not only is no bogy formed, and upon it no salutary dread which may act as a drag on her downward path superadded, but the patient has little or no saving sense of isolation and even no knowledge of many of her actions. The hysteric cannot inhibit because one must, of course, be conscious of an impending action before one can take any steps to prevent it.

Keeping then clearly in mind the normally wide range of the feminine mind-type, its

complexity and consequent tendency to instability, and knowing that it is subject, like the other type, to the same law of balance between its two parts (the individual and the common mind or common sense) for the maintenance of mental health and of mental comfort, we begin to understand how important it is that its possessor should above all things be brought up in surroundings that will secure the widest and freest human intercourse and contact with the outside world; that all the great principles of religion and morals which are fixed and serve as a final court of appeal within us should be early implanted and which, as founded on love, are readily absorbed by the feminine mind; that, in short, each and every of the faculties and instincts should be so developed that the individual, at the period of his or her real entry into the society of the world, should possess a well-stocked and wholesome common sense (common mind) fitted to deal with every ordinary and likely impression and idea, *i.e.*, with every item of the individual portion of the mind that may be brought to its notice.

Given a reasonably good heredity a feminine mind, thus wisely educated, will present to the world the very highest attainable type of mental development, a range of vision, a clearness of faith, a conception and love of ideals, a rapidity of perception, a breadth of judgment, a love and appreciation of the beautiful; all under the control of a reasoning power not slavishly tied to material possessions, never accepting the narrow and practical as the only view but beautifying by idealizing even the most carnal and sensual of our appetites. " A little lower than the angels" may this orderly type of the perfect feminine mind be styled; while, by way of contrast and comparison, it is hard to say more than " a little higher than the brute " of many of the pure specimens of the masculine mind, which, beyond some perfection of the mathematical faculty in its application to money, a certain regularity of action dependent on the same faculty, and a pertinacity and fidelity which it shares unequally with the bull-dog, has little or nothing to distinguish it from the higher animals, with which indeed, with much

HYSTERIA

persistence, it claims a distant relationship.

Please remember the absence of any sex line. Most men who achieve renown and inspire affection and respect, and all men of fine character, brilliancy or genius, have, if not the perfect feminine type of mind, a large admixture of it, whilst the comparative absence of masculine characteristics in the great majority of women is often discounted in our admiration and respect by a conspicuous weakness in some of the best attributes that belong exclusively to the feminine mind-type, and as the fall is greater the consequences are more evident and more deplorable.

And the great enemy to the formation of the perfect mind being in both types the Ego, and as woman by her very position in society, by the ingrained habit of centuries, by her surroundings, by suggestion ever ringing in her ears, and above all by her restriction to self-adornment in sexual competition, is by every artificial and natural means provoked to its magnification, it can be no matter for surprise if she thereby comes frequently to grief.

But apart from her special environment there are in women other causes at work that gravely endanger her mental stability. The question of mental balance is simple in a man; he has, as a rule, only his reasoning powers to bring into line with his individual propensities, but in the woman you have deep instincts firmly implanted in her that call for gratification. Take but the principal one, the maternity instinct, with all that it implies of unselfish love of the helpless, of a comfortable home of which she is mistress, of the companionship of, and reliance on, a mate. Here you have indeed a weight on one side of the balance, and if you cannot find the natural counterpoise, the gratification of the instinct, you will have indeed a hard task to find anything to put in place of it. The problem is complicated by the fact that being an instinct the possessor of it is unconscious, or but half conscious, of its possession and influence and cannot therefore readily help herself.

It would be easy to name other mental faculties, all instinctive in their character, that also frequently complicate the main-

HYSTERIA

tenance of balance in the feminine type of mind in both sexes.

The problem of balance therefore in the feminine type of mind, and in those persons whose mental constitution contains a considerable admixture of it, is one that calls for the most careful thought.

The great point is to understand it and in your calculations to adequately allow for it. Otherwise, you may very often be faced with a problem that seems insoluble, and may be tempted in a feeble manner to imitate the octopus in emptying your ink bag the better to conceal your discomfiture and retreat.

The better to obtain a clear picture of the situation it will be instructive to devote a short space to the effects, in other departments of life than medicine, of the misunderstandings and false situations that arise from the habit, dear to the masculine mind, of translating all phenomena, mental and physical, in terms of himself, and it must be remembered that this one-sided and false point of view is the outcome of the fact that, by reason of its concentration on the practical and material sides of life, the

masculine type has obtained the control of all the great political, legal and scientific systems and therefore holds at its sole discretion all the coercive powers, the military, naval and police, and most of the scientific, and a large share of the literary powers of the day.

Its standards are therefore the usually-accepted standards in all civil and military concerns, and, though it cannot bring under its dominion the spiritual side of man, it is engaged in an incessant warfare with it. Selecting from religion only those maxims, such as justice and truth, and, with one eye on the voting booths, the material side of charity, which suit its purpose and act as pillars and foundations to its plan, it rejects the wider spiritual view of charity, the real and original and only strict meaning of the term, the love of God and in the second place of your neighbour because he is a creature of God, so perverts this virtue into a socio-politico-material monstrosity that takes form in the workhouse, the relieving officer and the hospital, that truth, shrouding her keenest hits in proverbial form, has been provoked to the

HYSTERIA

satirical expression " as cold as charity."
The pure masculine type of mind with its
one talent, reason, but reason carefully
restricted in definition to its purely mathematical side in argument and its material
possessions and powers in evidence, puts an
unrelenting heel on every opponent, on
every advocate of wider, and presumably
higher, conceptions, runs the world and
throws a none too loving eye on the older
universities that are rightly suspected of
harbouring, in their theological and philo-
sophical faculties, a spirit of wider range
and establishing, as rivals to them, mere
examining institutions, and, when these are
discredited, modern universities in industrial
centres, in which it fondly hopes that the
material and the practical may hold almost
undisputed sway.

Because so much higher in constitution
and so much more prone to disintegration,
because so much more individual in
character and so much weaker in combination, the feminine mind-type, where mere
counting of heads decides the day, can make
but a poor fight, and while she pricks the
thick hide of the enemy with her keen rapier

of wit and satire, and holds him up to public ridicule by her subtlety of discernment, cannot secure the reins of power and therefore prove her capacity to mend the rents and tears in the garment of society. Have we not at the present moment three excellent examples of this strife of mind-types in the political and religious arenas! The Celt in Ireland, and even after years of residence in other lands, loathed and despised the material system adopted by England in her desire to assist him, just as he loathed her materialistic religion with its soup-kitchens and other venal temptations in times of famine, and, not comprehending the type of masculine mind that honestly considers the material as the only valuable and real, suspected all her best and purest motives, exalting above England's first statesmen the most gaseous degenerate of her own feminine type, provided he had wit and a certain speciousness; selecting often out of pure malice those which in her heart she least esteemed to represent her in Parliament so only that they might prove sharp thorns in the side of her enemy. But now that Irish self-government is within

HYSTERIA 103

sight the loudest threats are not heard from her feminine lips but from the masculine type resident in the North, who fear— perhaps without real cause — an attack on their money-bags and possessions, and yet Home Rule, if secured for Ireland, will have been done so only by her representatives having at length seen the wisdom of silence and of copying the ways and means of political success of Englishmen, typical of the purely masculine line of action: practical, practical, practical!!

And the Suffragist movement supplies an equally good and similar example. Like the Irish, the women in this country had a strong case in their demand that the feminine mind-type should be allowed some share in ruling the land they inhabited, and who shall justly grudge them some satisfaction of this claim when we remember how patiently they bore with the deprivation until the real danger to them of an extended male franchise, with its influx of low-class masculine type in large numbers, arose. Then woman spoke, but, like the Celt, quickly perceived that mere protest would secure no rapid success

and that her chance might be gone for many years if the male franchise were extended ere she secured the vote. Then she made the same mistake as the Celt. Instead of proceeding in the way that alone carries weight with the masculine mind, by silent combination and by strictly - reasoned speeches, she bubbled over and lost control of her more degenerate or less-balanced colleagues, always, as I have said, a large class in the feminine type, and emotion in its wilder forms and action of the most disorderly character, precisely as in the Irish situation, assumed that prominence loved by the hysterical, who cares nothing for its disastrous effect on a cause sustainable by many valid arguments and making a strong appeal to fair play, provided she is only well in the limelight. And the religious world furnishes us with a last parallel. Fifty years ago the Church of England was sunk in a lazy indifference, when her sleep was broken in upon by that truly feminine spirit, the ritualist movement, which taunted her with her betrayal of the real Christian spirit, parading before her indignant eyes some of the beautiful symbolic ceremony of

pre-Reformation days, reminding her insistently that her rubrics claimed continuity with the early and mediæval Church full of spirituality and self-denial, and lastly—worst cut of all—demonstrated, by the example of high-minded, self-sacrificing and devoted men, that higher ideals were still, as ever, capable of reaching and influencing for good the most hopeless and heart-broken of the human dust heap, and that poverty, humility and charity were more ennobling to the character than respectability and material possessions though located in the seats of the mighty. Even the Bashi-Bazouks of the campaign, who, as in the Irish and Suffragist movements, were of course early on the scene and did much to embarrass it by their hysterical antics and their unrestrained language, could not arrest its current, which has now attained such volume as to sweep nearly all that represents the old masculine type of mind in the Church of England away. And the result has not been what was confidently predicted of it, a splitting up of the Church, but rather a re-welding together of an old fabric that was tending by neglect to fall into ruin, a

rebreathing of a better spirit into dry bones.

Personally I may be allowed to explain that I am by conviction a strong anti in regard to the questions of Home Rule, Female Suffrage and Anglicanism in any shape, but this does not hinder me from fairly stating the pro-case as I conceive it, conscious as I am that the Almighty Dollar and the mere gratification of our senses, our present chief standards of success, are unworthy and base, and hoping that, by a fresh infusion of mind, our ideals may be elevated and a wider and a better outlook secured for humanity; and we may be fortified in the face of possible fears by what science and philosophy tell us, that all the phenomena of life and nature are but the pieces of a puzzle partly broken up and rearranged by successive generations as new facts are discovered and wider combinations attained, and that each reconstructed puzzle is confidently viewed as the one real and final solution.

I have endeavoured to give in a pictorial way an idea of the feminine mind-type, and if only the reader can gather from my

HYSTERIA

description of its many and elusive elements a fair general conception of its whole he will find the study of its derangements, which has puzzled many, quite easy to follow and to comprehend.

CHAPTER VII

HYSTERIA

i.e., the loss of balance in the feminine type of mind

PART II.—THE SYMPTOMS AND TREATMENT OF HYSTERIA

Special predisposing influences in the production of Hysteria

THESE may all be grouped under two headings, which for simplicity I will call the *exalted Ego*, meaning thereby all that tends to over-cultivation of self, and the *starved instinct*, which includes all checks to the proper gratification of normal instincts, for such are the two great underlying causes of every hysterical development.

We must, however, also make allowance for three different types of feminine mind commonly met with, which we may thus classify:

(1) *The pure feminine mind-type*. Though occasionally men, and very charming ones, fall under this heading, it contains, as we should expect, a high percentage of women, and may therefore be spoken of in the femi-

HYSTERIA

nine gender. Femininity is apparent in all her works and ways; she is a real "female woman" ever and everywhere.

(2) *The weak feminine mind-type*, a product often of unstable mental heredity, in which the balance is visibly unsteady. Many men belong to this class.

(3) *The mixed type*, having many properties of the masculine mind. The ordinary Englishwoman and the business French and Belgian woman may be regarded as fair examples of it.

Now each one of these three classes will react very differently in similar circumstance. The first will be stable in her very instability, exhibiting in ordinary life, by the active play of her emotions, the oscillations of a sensitive balance tending to re-equilibration; but under gross and prolonged mismanagement, or under some severe or sudden check to some one of her deep instincts, such as love, may be expected to exhibit the widest functional perversions, the most perfect example of the disorder in its fullest range, the Hysteria major or malignant Hysteria of the text-books. *The second type*, a very large one, weak from

the start, and reacting to the ordinary stimuli of life always abnormally; essentially unstable during her whole life, excitable, weakly emotional, selfish, indolent, unless goaded to exertion by the lure of self-gratification; always ailing and sick because her various organs, for want of regularized nerve control, are ever at fault in their functional duties; receptive to any idea that can titivate her emotions, throwing herself literally into each new movement in which she sees a new mental stimulant; unable to be straightforward but exaggerating and colouring her every statement, unreliable and untruthful; of shallow intellect but often smart and quick by fits and starts, she forms the backbone of every anti-movement, of every fad, of every new system, and specially delights in those that have a trace of sexual piquancy. We are all familiar with the type, and most of all can recognize it at a glance by certain physical characteristics. It is from this type that the largest number of Hysterics are recruited; they do not often rise to great heights even in this disorder but are rarely for long free altogether from some taint of it. *The*

third type comprises the great bulk of ordinary middle and lower-class Englishwomen, slow in thought, safe from temptation because void of imagination, adopting the current standards without concern for any great principles, unambitious and docile, good mothers, and generally pattern wives, steady and, above all, reliable because mentally the most stable of the three types. In this class may be ranged quite a considerable number of males who, under the stimulus of a wider life than that of women, exhibit often artistic taste and skill of a high order. It is the women belonging to this class who alone of their sex are fitted to battle with the world and compete with men in the duties of life that call for steady application to uninteresting and routine work, and unless under the sense of grave disappointment, or handicapped by the times of stress that belong specially to their sex, they rarely fall victims to any serious form of Hysteria. In all women the menstrual cycle tends somewhat to lower the standard of stability, though too much of this has been made as a factor, and indeed it is open to question whether its effect has not been

increased by the attention paid to it by the medical profession and by the quite unnecessary precautions recommended at such times in the case of the average woman. The same applies to puberty and the climacteric. If women were left more alone in these matters, and only the real organic diseases treated when necessary by surgical procedure, as is the case with men, it is certain that, beyond those blights of frustrated maternal function called fibroid tumours, and the disorders which follow on infections, that the law should do more to render impossible, a long list of disorders peculiar to women would disappear from the world. An immense improvement in this respect has taken place within my memory, but superstitions die hard and many a woman's life is still wrecked by her attention being wrongly concentrated on the sexual apparatus, and the result is seen in the Nemesis that waits on self-concentration—Hysteria. She does not become immoral, but morbid. The most scathing condemnation of such malpractice I have ever heard came from the lips of one of the greatest medical experts in this special department

HYSTERIA

at the present day. Too much so-called sexual physiology as a subject of instruction for young girls is also to be strongly deprecated as tending in the same direction, and one has only to read the advertisement columns, especially of some of the pseudo-religious prints of the day, to see that there are, as we saw was the case in young men, plenty of vampires ready to magnify a function into a mystery and to batten on this special form of anxiety, though the Book which they expound with so much unction wisely refers the sex to " the law of her mother and the covenant of her God" as the surest of guides.

Hysteria: What it is and what it is not.—
Emotion, even if it appear to the more phlegmatic to be in excess, is not Hysteria, for in many persons of both sexes who are perfectly stable, the natural outlet to the strain of adverse circumstances takes the form of tears, sobs, prolonged laughter, tremors and other muscular actions, flushing or great volubility. Nor under great provocation should a convulsion, or even a succession of them, be thus branded but be read as a physiological effort to restore the

mental equilibrium on the natural lines of least resistance and proof only of a healthy tendency in a sensitive nature even if they occasionally pass beyond voluntary control; for there is no fixed boundary in Nature between health and functional disorder, the first is physiology in normal circumstances, the second physiology in abnormal ones, and both have one common goal, the maintenance of life. But nevertheless we shall be safe in adopting as a general rule that all symptoms beyond our conscious and voluntary self-control are those of disease and apply this rule to Hysteria.

The Symptoms of Hysteria.—The feminine mind-type being in its fullest development co-relative with the whole brain, the signs and evidence of its disorder will be co-terminous with the body, each organ whereof is represented in some part of the brain by a centre of direction. The list of symptoms will be therefore necessarily a very extensive one, and, to prevent confusion, the best plan will be to consider in broad groups the main psychical functions and give instances of their perversions.

The higher brain is of course an artificial

HYSTERIA

division, for we have no certain data on which to found any strict boundaries, but we may understand by the term that part of the brain that is *en rapport* with conscious thought. Perversions of consciousness are very common in Hysteria, and indeed it may be said that every case of real Hysteria involves some impairment of it, and the interesting and often-debated question therefore presents itself: Are Hysterics fully responsible for their thoughts and apparently voluntary actions? And the answer is: Control of them is always weak and often apparently wanting. The same is true of their memory regarding them. Then is not Hysteria a form of Insanity? The dividing line in bad cases is a fine one, but there is such a line, and if you carefully study a severe case you will find that the mental balance is never in Hysteria " off the pivot," as in Insanity, and that the oscillations, though so vigorous and rapid as scarcely to be followed by the observer, are nevertheless present and, though they lack rhythm and equality, are, as always, sure evidence that the jeopardized balance is still in working order. And one of the best

proofs of this fact is that recovery may take place quite suddenly even in the most violent of attacks, a phenomenon never seen—or seen so very rarely as not to invalidate the rule—in Insanity. There therefore always remains in Hysteria some control power in the higher mind, some consciousness and some memory, however dim, and even in those cases in which the Psyche, as it is called, is split up, when each hemisphere of the brain appears to act independently of the other, and when the patient asserts that each half constitutes an entirely independent self, you will, on careful examination, find proof of it. I knew some twenty years ago a lady who while talking, reciting or playing could simultaneously write a good and original essay on any selected subject, and this without looking at the writing hand, which did its work equally well on a pad placed on or under the table at which this lady was seated. She said that the writing was beyond her control. Much of it was emotional and foolish, and parts distinctly obscene, showing that some of the lower instinctive mental faculties were at work. One manuscript was a false and lurid account of a parturition

HYSTERIA

(the lady was young, single and of blameless life), with illustrations of terrible hooked instruments with spear points; the whole production very realistic. When I suggested that circlets should be added to complete the picture, a series of large connecting rings was automatically added. This patient also claimed the power to throw herself into a cataleptic state, and in that condition to be able to send her soul on errands of inquiry into the past and future. The result of any information thus obtained consisted only of vague generalities that might fit almost any case, or be adapted to it, no clearer details in the way of a test for truth being ever obtainable. One could not fail to remark how eagerly even intelligent members of the audience sought to adapt the predictions and statements to themselves or their friends, and how unpopular it was to be critical. This lady did not use her powers for purposes of making money and only for the kudos it brought her.

I have also frequently witnessed in hysterical persons instances of pseudo-double personality, two very opposite

rôles in life being played in succession, but this was never the real dual personality of psychic forms of Epilepsy, for the patient could always be recalled to her former self promptly by some simple means.

In cataleptic states the appearance of the patient may be so changed as to be scarcely recognizable. Generally there is great pallor, with large immovable pupils, a cadaveric rigidity of the facial muscles with slowing of the heart and the respirations; in fact, both the latter may appear to be on the point of cessation. All the vital functions seem lowered, and one can well understand how long periods of fasting with but slight diminution of weight are possible in these mental states.

The results of these exhibitions on the patient herself are harmful, and the tendency to instability increases markedly by repetition, so that at last a look, a word, or ten drops of Indian hemp in water, is sufficient to induce the scene. We cannot, however, linger over this very interesting subject, instances of which are of common occurrence

and objects of surprise to non-medical and wonder-seeking onlookers; yet even the most sympathetic of observers cannot help being often shocked by what must seem to be intentional deception so unwisely and unnecessarily added to phenomena remarkable enough in themselves and they naturally ask the question: " Why this moral obliquity? May not the whole demonstration have been carefully studied and rehearsed with the sole view to deception?" The correct answer is to be probably found in a study of the *mental equation* (see Chapter IX), and in the conscious resistance to some one of the moral faculties having fallen with a corresponding rise in others, and to view the matter thus pictorially will help us to visualize what otherwise could be expressed only in abstract terms. It gives us a percept instead of a concept.

The middle brain, again a division not meant to be anatomical, the *pied-à-terre* of the subconscious or subliminal mind, the seat of the instincts and the habits, sometimes called the " acquired reflexes," next concerns us, and a host of dis-

orders of many shades is rendered possible by its perversions from the normal. In comparison with the higher brain it is subject in health to fewer oscillations, for the impressions it directly receives are less in number. The sexual instinct, which in women is mainly maternal in hue, shows curious and sometimes revolting alterations, but of such a matter it suffices us to say that their direction is not towards open vice but to psychical exaltations of the sex instinct, with which certain practices are sometimes combined, and in connection with which we may often acquit the victim of any knowledge of conscious wrong. The perverted maternity instinct is seen in an extreme devotion to animals, or even to inanimate objects, and in the various ways of "mothering," in a weak, silly manner and productive of little good, the heathen, the drunkard, and especially the vicious who are its objects, often harming them and bringing ridicule upon otherwise lofty causes. Other instincts, such as the artistic, may undergo similar aberration with deterioration or improvement in ability, and I have known a mere dauber become converted

HYSTERIA

into a painter of considerable taste and merit when suffering from a severe general form of Hysteria. There is practically no limit to the strange phenomena that may be seen when this same subconscious mind is perturbed. It may then throw to the surface words, expressions and conceptions that lay buried therein, or make its oscillations the basis—as I have explained in Chapter VI—of endless mimicries of disease. The habits or acquired reflexes exhibit a like disorder and may be broken up, combined in fantastic fashion, or, for the time being, obliterated; the methodical man or woman may become careless of time and place,—night as the time of wakefulness and activity may be substituted for day—and a confirmed smoker, or even opium-eater, may absolutely forget the existence of these narcotics. I have known instances of all. There is no hard-and-fast line in Hysteria as there are no real frontiers in the brain, and all sorts and varieties of disorder may be mingled together in one single hysterical individual, the conscious mind, as I have said, being always one of the parties to it. Occasionally, however, what may look like isolated

hysterical symptoms appear, and these are always the most puzzling to the physician. I can recall a highly-emotional man who had the " gift of tongues." If he met with opposition in any cherished design, or were influenced by suggestion in any form, he would forthwith deliver himself of a stream of gibberish which varied on each occasion and had a specious resemblance to language, by the emphasis and modulation given to parts of it. He would argue in it or preach in it. It contained many Latin and Greek words, and yet he professed an entire ignorance of both those tongues. He was not insane, and explained the process by saying that he felt an irresistible impulse to act as he did, but his flow of speech could always be arrested by loud laughter or ridicule from his audience, or by any sudden and, to him, impressive incident. Eventually he lost the " gift," but was left with an impulse to it, which he could restrain, whenever anything upset him gravely. He was always a copious shedder of tears on the least provocation, and equally on occasions of joy, sorrow or anger.

HYSTERIA

The lower brain and spinal cord and sympathetic centres, that are in psychic relationship with the function of organs and their secretions and excretions, with the control of the blood supply, the many functions of the skin, the rhythmic movements of the heart and lungs, and the peristaltic movement of the intestines, make up our last grouping. Disturbances by excess or diminution may occur in any one or more of them, and may be restricted to them or accompanied by evidences of Hysteria in higher centres. Perhaps an example best appreciated by the laity is seen in the case of the liver. I knew an hysterical woman who in any opposition to her special form of self-esteem invariably developed jaundice, and not only was the output of bile into the bowel brought to a standstill but the actual amount secreted by the liver was much reduced. Another lady, who nourished herself on the sympathies that attach to invalidism, told me that her heart was so weak that the ascent of the smallest hill brought on palpitation and irregular action, and this was, as I found, an actual result. One day I took her after dark up a hill, the

slope of which was obscured by the darkness and conversation, and her heart remained quite unaffected, but when told of the ruse next day it became at once so disordered that her friends requested me, for the sake of their own comfort, not again to try such an experiment. I have seen a sharp attack of spasmodic asthma follow immediately on a wound to the self-love. Great exaggeration of the muscular reflexes is a general accompaniment of Hysteria, but again they may be decreased almost to the point of extinction. Great dilatation of the pupils of the eye and failure of reflex response to light or distance are not unfrequently seen, and sometimes the pupils may become unequal on the two sides or ovoid in shape. Perhaps the most astounding of phenomena is one that has been witnessed in more than one hospital; a reversal of direction in the peristaltic muscular action of the coats of the intestine, which in health gradually works food slowly through the coils of bowel towards the outlet; while reversal of this direction occurs only in complete stoppage and, when unrelieved, is accompanied by another and grave symptom, fæcal vomiting.

HYSTERIA

But Hysteria has provided a parallel even to this. Not long ago in an East-end hospital there resided a patient who had on three previous occasions, by reason of these symptoms, undergone operations, nothing wrong being found in any of them, and she was prepared to again submit to a like procedure; but her past history having come to life she was saved from the experience and recovered. Now it is hardly conceivable that any element of fraud could have been present in this case, nothing was to be gained by facing a grave surgical risk. But, on the other hand, and about the same time, but in another hospital, a woman, recognized as a victim to Hysteria in many shapes, had also fæcal vomiting, but on careful observation she was discovered to be artificially bringing about the process; yet even in this case, knowing the possible wide variations in the mental equation seen in Hysteria and the horrible procedure to which she had recourse, it may fairly be doubted whether the imposture was as consciously deliberate as it appears, for the moral sense is always blunted in Hysteria, and there is an absence of shame on exposure

such as is never witnessed in similar people in health. Let me then ere we leave the question of Hysteria once more ask the reader to pause before he thoughtlessly ascribes Insanity or fraud to any hysteric case. However grave the symptom in Hysteria, it can be stopped at once by some sufficiently strong counter-emotion, and if either of the women with fæcal vomiting had been told that a favourite child was lying at home in danger of death the vomiting would almost certainly have ceased and the patient forthwith have re-found the power of returning to her home; but remember carefully it must be an *abnormally strong* counteracting emotion, whereas, in a normal state of mental health, sufficient inducement to recovery in emotional states would have been found in some *common and everyday emotion ;* while in Insanity no emotion, however powerful, would have any effect. The difference in the three situations is therefore a very real one and must be kept in mind.

The foregoing is intended not as a detailed description of Hysteria in its protean shapes but more as an effort to provide a mental

HYSTERIA

chart of the disorder so that the reader can obtain and retain a clear view of the action of the laws that underlie Hysteria and upon the effects of which its symptoms are founded.

CHAPTER VIII

HYSTERIA

i.e., loss of balance in the feminine type of mind

PART III.—THE TREATMENT OF HYSTERIA

THE treatment of Hysteria is a battle but not on the solid earth, a combat of minds between patient and adviser, and the weapons of the latter are not those of the pharmacy nor of science, for these must be kept carefully in the background and reserved as mechanical aids after the real victory has been secured, as props and stays on the stony road that has to be travelled after the patient is on her feet and before she can walk with assurance on the broad highway of humanity. Therefore the first essential to success is to:

(1) *Understand and control the patient.* Not only is it necessary to get on good terms with the patient—that is easily effected, for she will at first regard you as a probable ally, as one to become in the near future a

HYSTERIA

follower in her train—the first look she throws at you under half-shut lids, and with eyes that affect to be tired and indifferent, is but the first stage in that " summing up " of you which, translated into words, would often take some such form as this: " Another ass that thinks he is going to control me; we shall see! " But the doctor must not, in foolish self-assurance, despise the enemy, an attitude so often assumed and about which the patient is sure to be informed however far from the sick-room it may be expressed, whether in signs or words. Like a skilful gambler the doctor's look must conceal his thoughts, and at the earliest opportunity, and after he has made himself master of all necessary details from friends, who rarely or never can give any useful clue to the mystery, he should dismiss the latter to have a heart-to-heart talk with the patient. Now, and just in proportion to his knowledge and skill, he will obtain real information. No real active organic disease will be found, for as in Neurasthenia so in Hysteria all the vagaries seen are but the oscillations of a healthy mind in a state of stress and blindly seeking a balance, and

would vanish of their own accord in face of tangible disease. Some quiescent organic mischief, having no part in the production of the present symptoms, may be found, but even this is rare, while, almost invariably, some trivial displacement of a kidney or uterus, ovary or stomach, or some functional derangement, evidenced by headache, flatulency, etc., will be brought with great formality to the doctor's notice, and he will be told—and not truthfully—that Dr So-and-so considered it a most important disease, one that would take years to cure and which required the utmost care and attention if death itself, or chronic invalidity, were not to be the result. The wise man will not contradict, still less will he remark that such-and-such an organ could be stitched into position by surgical operation, for unlike the Neurasthenic, who has the practical mind and dreads operations, because he fears the possible consequences, the Hysteric would promptly fall in with the suggestion and, even if the doctor failed to carry it out, he would find himself for ever quoted as an authority, and styled an expert or specialist, who strongly advised a serious

HYSTERIA

operation as the one and only cure, and who, but for the fact that she (the patient) was at death's door at that time, would at once have performed it. For a marked characteristic of the hysterical mind is that it has pluck, if courage can be ascribed to one who lives mainly for the sympathies of the day and has little thought, or fear, of the morrow. The doctor's next step is, under assurance of the strictest secrecy (which he must most honourably observe both in the spirit and in the letter), to obtain from the patient a real and complete mental history, showing by his intercalated observations that he fully understands and can sympathize with all her grievances and contrarieties, and that he reckons none of them as trivial since they are of importance to her; the real test. If the doctor be himself in the widest sense a man of understanding he will rarely fail to get the whole truth, and the picture thus obtained will be very dissimilar to that which even the nearest and dearest of the patient's friends would ever have dreamt of. He will hear of cherished desires frustrated, secret ambitions balked, keen emotions and feelings

chilled; in short, he will see that the patient *has been misunderstood*, no silly phrase but one representing the real and deep wound of a sensitive and often a really high and fine nature whose legitimate and normal Ego has been dwarfed, and her instincts starved or blighted. He will, further, be astonished to find that the patient, if she meets a kindred, or at least a comprehending, soul, can be truthful, and that her deceit and lack of truth previously noted is but what she conceived as necessary to play the only *rôle* left her in life—that of a debilitated and sympathy-craving invalid. "Tout comprendre est tout pardonner," and in the doctor's case one may often add "tout pouvoir." How extraordinary is such a confession; what a totally different person and character you have presented to view, and if you shut your eyes the better to construct your mental picture you may be startled on again opening them at the contrast that presents itself. How little we really know of human life, and how far it is from the picture that casual and even intimate observation often provides for us, though it would obviously never do to wear

HYSTERIA

always one's real mind or heart on one's sleeve; and even if we did, it would only be our mind as viewed and appraised by itself.

One cheering result I have gained from such disclosures is the conviction that there are few intentionally and maliciously bad people in the world, but there are a host of weak and feeble persons, and that very few of them have any compass that points to any definite magnetic north; conventions, bitterly hated by many a woman who outwardly affects to worship them, there are in plenty, and some feeble principles, mere wisps of thought touched by a faint hope as by a sun ray, and chiefly used as counters in the game of life. Instincts deep and broad there are which, controlled and guided by the reason and allowed due gratification, could make life sane and tolerable, but to make it consistent, satisfying to the higher mind, and occasionally really happy, you must have much more: an unshakable conviction that there is an end in which the soul can rest with every longing satisfied and every inequality of life made straight. Science cannot fill the gap; she starts with a nescio

and ends of necessity with the same; her duty being confined to the reduction of phenomena to the order that best fits the Zeitgeist, the simplification of a problem not its solution, and the *rôle* of philosophy is to co-ordinate her conclusions into wider generalizations. Both are of inestimable use as training-grounds for the mind, but neither makes any pretence of a final definition.

To say more would be to exceed the limits of my subject and my remarks are merely the thoughts that must arise in all reflecting minds brought face to face with the problems of life as set by the nude mind; and it is not for the doctor to do more than quietly regret this absence in the life of sufferers of any guiding star that would be of assistance to him in giving direction to his efforts. Indeed, not long ago a chronic Hysteric rose from her bed and interested herself again in life at the instigation of Christian science, and a lady in the north of London, after years spent as an invalid with hysterical paralysis of both legs, was in a few minutes cured by a revivalist preacher who had taken up faith-healing. She heard

HYSTERIA

of his powers, was impressed, sent for him and was cured. These cases show the profound influence even of very third-rate ideals on minds not necessarily of small calibre but untrained in habits of clear thought, and I was most careful to offer no opposition in either case; a half loaf being not only better than no bread but the quantity often better suited to a feeble digestion. As to the result. It was durable in the first and not in the second patient, who could not be made to comprehend, when the pastor subsequently proved to be morally a friable vessel, that such fact had nothing whatever to do with herself, and that a leper may show you the right road though he has not the strength himself to walk along it.

The question of all mental treatment is so important, and the subject so interesting, that a strong temptation to extend the theme arises in my mind, but I feel that sufficient has been said to give all that I can here pretend to supply; the direction in which treatment to be successful should be carried out, with the one objective before the mind, the restoration of the patient to

normal life and activity. One fallacy—dear to the masculine mind and afforded a prominent place in many an official textbook—I wish to condemn, namely, that the deprivation of sexual congress is the great if not the only thorn in the flesh of the sufferer and the one which incessantly vexes and disturbs her spirit. In fact, more than one writer goes so far as to say that the thoughts connected therewith are to be screwed out of her by hypnotism, or other form of suggestion, and met by the installation in her mind of negative ideas; and if these statements are disputed one is met by the remark, " Oh, you can't deny the truth for the patient herself acknowledges it." Quite so, it is precisely the idea that an Hysteric would concur in, just as she concurred with Dr Charcot in his acceptance of the idea that disease could be transmitted by a magnet or even by a glass of water. " Fooling him to the top of his bent " is precisely the game of games for her, why I know not, unless it be that she thereby expresses her contempt for the masculine type of mind and her insight into some of its inherent weaknesses. Marriage doubtless

HYSTERIA

often cures a woman, but chiefly by responding to the demand of her instincts for unselfish love with its idea of self-immolation, but any want of response to affection will bring a relapse into Hysteria even after marriage. Maternity is the best cure of all. There are few women, outside the ranks of the degenerate and perverted, to whom crude sensuality alone is a potent appeal, though most women are quite willing that men should believe the contrary, and bad ones of every grade encourage the idea because their profit arises from this misunderstanding, while among intimates they laugh heartily at it all the time. That there is a vein of weak psychic immorality in many types of Hysteria one cannot help recognizing, but this is as a rule shrouded in noble sentiments that doubtless are regarded as its excuse or justification. As evidence that this disorder cannot usually have sensual gratification as its chief foundation, I may add that, for a series of years, I attended several communities of religious women, and amongst them never witnessed any trace of Hysteria; and this also I find is the experience of other doctors, even in silent

and purely contemplative orders who are not engaged in active outdoor work, and I am certain therefore that a well-directed, pure and high type of love amply suffices to meet all the instinctive requirements of the order to which I refer. Not only is Hysteria rare in nuns, but amongst no other class of women have I known such gaiety, content and generally sound mental and physical equilibrium.

Having then first of all secured a perfect picture of the patient's mind, of her real self, the doctor's aim will be to sketch a path along which she can safely travel towards health, and as a first step thereto he will seek:

(2) *To alter her surroundings* to her benefit. Friends, books, rooms, medicines, everything and everyone have been moulded by the patient to serve as supports of, and a setting to, her state of invalidism, and all have become, in consequence, active agents of suggestion. This atmosphere must be changed. The patient's muscles are weak from want of exercise, her digestion enfeebled by misuse, her mind restricted in range and concentrated on trivialities; in short, the

HYSTERIA

difficulties seem to be almost unsurmountable, and yet as both mind and body are in constitution sound, both will be found to have retained their elasticity and capability of a rebound to health and vigour if only the suggestive obstacles thereto can be removed. And here one of the sanest methods, that of Dr Weir Mitchell, comes to our aid. Its drawbacks are its quite unnecessary expense and the measure of discredit that has accrued to it from its application to unsuitable cases. Probably its novelty was for a time its greatest asset, for it has dropped considerably out of a favour which it did much to deserve. A grasp of the situation, common sense, a wise sympathy and gentle firmness, are the virtues of an efficient Weir-Mitchell nurse, for she is the great agent of cure. Visitors and letters and all exciting outside news are taboo for the first week or more, according to the patient's conditions and needs. The doctor himself is often best out of sight, available at call if both nurse and patient agree in wishing to see him, but not unless, if everything is going well. I need not enter into details as to diet; this should be

a very full one in the emaciated and restricted but varied in the corpulent. Simple or galvanic massage of the forehead and back of the neck late in the evening is a useful aid to repose. If that fail, the general hot pack or the local hot pack over the stomach should be resorted to. Real insomnia is not common, but in cases in which it is of occasional recurrence, and a source of trouble, I recommend a plan which I have found a specific for persons endowed with a vivid imagination. I simply instruct the patient how to tell herself, silently, a story. This story is reserved only as an inducement to sleep; any theme that interests her may be selected, and she herself should be the central figure. In a week or less, a habit of picking up the story at the point at which it was dropped and continuing it, is developed, and the patient soon becomes thoroughly interested in the various fancied situations that arise. I know many not hysterical sufferers who have used this simple plan for years, and who, once they have picked up the thread of their story, fall asleep in a very short time; it acts, moreover, by keeping all disturbing

HYSTERIA

and unpleasant thoughts out of the mind. I find in men that military campaigns are selected as the favourite subject, and the same story in its various developments may extend over years. A much-worried business man wrote to say that he had followed my plan for fifteen years and that he felt sure that it alone had kept him out of the asylum, and though absolutely incredulous at first even as to its possibility, he had found it easy and pleasant after a short perseverance. I adopted it for patients as a cure for sleeplessness thirty years ago, after remarking its utility in a highly-nervous family of children, and I have since found that story-telling aloud or to oneself is quite in familiar use as a sleep-producer in many nurseries. It is instructive to remark that, while the worst cases of Hysteria can and do avail themselves of the system, I have never known an insane person capable of doing so.

The strict Weir-Mitchell system may be relaxed as the patient improves, but a mere increase in weight—often regarded as positive proof of a cure—must not in itself be taken as an advancement, for the cure of

the mind is the great object in view and this must be directed towards some form of activity suitable and possible to the patient's age and social status. Often one of the colonies may be used as a lure, but the doctor should never advise at random, but obtain, if he does not possess it, a sure and certain knowledge of the suitability of any place recommended and necessary introductions, etc., for the patient.

Many cases of Hysteria occur among the working classes, generally in men after an accident that has frightened them severely. They are not malingerers; the paralysis—for that is the form in which it is generally seen—is real and beyond the control of the will-power, though still only functional. It is produced by the suggestion that severe injury has resulted from the accident, and is matured by the sympathies and suggestive allusions of neighbours. I have seen many bad instances of it. Here also it is essential to alter the surroundings of the patient and to assure him of his ability ere long to return to work, an end which the patient himself is often most desirous of attaining.

HYSTERIA

(3) *Endeavour to find systematic employment for the mind.* If you have carried out the first of my recommendations and really know the natural bent of her mind—and without this you will effect nothing at all—you are in a position to advise with effect. A child, even an adopted one if need be, for the childless is a sovereign remedy. For the woman who craves for marriage and the sympathy and love that attend it, a place in some colony which will give her a wider world to live in and a better opportunity to marry than in England. For the woman tied to routine house duties and unmarried, some outdoor work is best, for home industries are bad. For the woman with a little money and some adaptability the stage is one of the very best of employments. I shall never forget the case of a young lady of small income with inveterate Hysteria, who, on her parents' death, took up that profession, and how quickly it made a cheerful, healthy and young woman out of a worn and sickly-looking invalid. I need not give a list of possible occupations, but only say that they should be such as the patient feels specially drawn to and that

offer a decent remuneration for work done. Let not the silly bogy of nervous breakdown obstruct anyone. In reality the hysterical woman is a little too full of nervous energy which only wants direction into useful and desirable channels to produce excellent fruit; and the doctor may safely assure doubting relatives and friends that he will cheerfully take all risks if the patient will follow his advice strictly and will persevere.

The above remarks apply to the still young and vigorous Hysteric, such as have not wilted through the years till they have become so irrevocably crooked, selfish and self-absorbed as to seem beyond the reach of any mental remedy; yet even of these some recover. The most hopeless of all are the wealthy and elderly spinsters whose susceptibilities none of their entourage dares to offend; but even for them the doctor who will not play the *rôle* of a mere parasite can often do more than he at first thinks possible; for behind all their mental and physical obliquities more of discernment and judgment may remain than the casual onlooker would give credit for. I recall such

HYSTERIA

a chronic case of inveterate Hysteria, in which the patient announced the onset of a new disease by telegram at intervals of every few days, and who, in his (for the sex was male) intervals of relief from functional paralysis, would, to excite attention and sympathy, go into the garden and bah like a sheep, or plaintively mew like a kitten, or shower pebbles on the neighbours' windows. He had summoned from London at various times every physician of name to minister to his symptoms, and always listened with apparent appreciation to their soothing platitudes, though he never took a dose of their physic nor followed one of their rules. To him, in my absence from town and by inadvertence, a very clever young surgeon was sent who, after a careful examination and a subsequent ink sketch of the organs with the handle of a pen on the patient's abdomen, replied to the usual question, " Now, what is your opinion of me? " with " You are the d——est fool I have seen for a long time." Instead of taking offence at this observation, the patient appreciated it, and long after used laughingly to say, " That is the most honest man I have ever

seen, though of course one could not live long on terms of the d——est fool with anyone." I do not cite this example as any commendation of either the attitude of mind, or the special language, adopted by the surgeon, but to show that, in the worst cases, there is usually, though in quiescence, a certain sanity of observation which it should be the doctor's aim to bring to the surface for use as his chief agent in the permanent cure of the invalid. In this case it was possible not only to do so, but to play also upon the patient's love of wealth and of financial reputation, and thus gradually to wean him from the state of abject self-concentration into which he, a really capable man, had gradually sunk from taking the wrong road at the commencement of his disorder; in this case by retiring from active work in the City in order to make himself a literary reputation, a line recommended to him, because he had suffered from " globus hystericus " as a result of a sharp disappointment.

I have always found it of the greatest advantage to address the hysterical sufferer, with whom I have established good terms,

HYSTERIA

from whom I have obtained a real life history, on the plane of his or her sound and actual self, and not on that of his or her hysterical and false personality. To explain and emphasize this most important point let us take a supposititious case: "A" has been in bed for two years with a "phantom abdominal tumour," areas of skin insensibility and bouts of hysterical vomiting, living in an atmosphere of pity and crowned with the halo of martyrdom. You have elicited the real history, and know the causes underlying it, and have agreed with the patient to "keep up appearances" with her friends for the present, but to work in conjunction with her for the satisfaction of what you know to be her special ambitions and desires; you have convinced her that you do not regard her as a malingerer and that you recognize clearly that her symptoms, though functional, are actual experiences to herself and beyond her power, by any simple act of good-will, to banish; that you have decided to place her in circumstances that will cease to hypnotize her and confirm her in the present disorder, and that when, by

such measures and aided by her collaboration, she has obtained efficient self-control, you will do your best to arrange that her life shall in future be adapted to the natural calls of her mind, to her instincts, her ambitions and her special capacities. Now, having established this most desirable mutual understanding, you must no longer treat her, when alone, as an hysterical invalid, but on the same level as you would a patient with a broken limb, an attack of broncho-pneumonia, or other temporary ailment which is sure to get better, and discuss the plans for her future advancement and success in life; not ignoring completely the tumour or vomiting, but referring to them as present inconveniences that are certain to pass away spontaneously as she becomes more normal.

In short, as you are conspiring together to help her out of a mental prison, your conversation should naturally turn on the pleasures of liberty.

The foregoing recommendation, though not in any treatise in Hysteria that I know of, is not a trivial one, but I think recommends itself to sound judgment and com-

HYSTERIA

mon sense and is the outcome of a long practical experience. Its one aim is to extract all that is mentally good and sound in the patient, and to build up on that foundation a new and healthy mental life.

(4) *Dramatic mental appeals and suggestions.* These sudden appeals to the imagination of the patient are rarely in the power of the doctor to command or to make use of. Faith cures, hypnotism, etc., are of this class, and the setting is as necessary, even more so, than the actual procedure. Thus, if you decide to avail yourself of any one of them, you must look to it that there is as large an audience as possible and that the *réclame* to follow shall be loud and far-reaching. Personally, I have always fought shy of them, while never opposing the patient's inclination if it be firmly set on the trial, for the proportion of temporary successes is small, and that of permanent cures even less, since you cannot often keep up the effect when you have secured it.

A typical " bed case " of several years' duration went, in charge of a doctor, to

Nancy to undergo a course of hypnotism. The enthusiasm of her companion, and the novelty of the situation and of the treatment, brought about so much improvement that she spent a subsequent month alone at a bright seaside home, walking about and apparently well. She was, later on, brought back to her own house by the doctor, looking remarkably well and walking with confidence, for her Hysteria had taken the form of paralysis of both legs. After the doctor's departure she returned to her room and bed within an hour, and to my knowledge remained there for several years, in spite of every effort to again rouse her to activity. These brilliant cures effected by hypnotism rarely stand the wear and tear even of a sheltered normal life, for the want of any system of following them up, any subsequent systematic adaptation to their environment, and it must never be forgotten that no Hysteric who is not fitted by treatment to respond to the *normal stimuli* of life, *i.e.*, to the ordinary conditions of life, can be regarded as cured. That is the only real test of recovery and nothing in the way of cure can be accepted in place of it. The

HYSTERIA

truth of this is before our eyes in the analogous condition of Alcoholism, which, like Hysteria, has in many cases a real and distinctive mental origin and dependence. The inebriates' reformatories have proved a failure in the experience of those very practical judges, the London police magistrates, and even a three years' residence therein has resulted in failure, although, as I am assured by keen observers who have had charge of such institutions, the inmate had absolutely lost all temptation to take alcohol and all craving for its exciting effect for at least a year prior to her release; and could she only have been kept under some supervision when outside, provided with easy work and sheltered—as she was when in the institution—from the worries and anxieties of life, she would certainly have experienced no difficulty in a lifelong abstinence. One system of cure for Alcoholism must be referred to, for it has proved itself a success in America—and I do not give the name because I do not wish to advertise it—by wisely founding its plan upon a knowledge of human nature. First of all, it possesses an alluring name.

Secondly, it impresses the patient further by allowing him when in the home to order and drink what alcohol he chooses, assuring him at the same time that the " cure " is so certain that it will succeed, in spite of everything, in eradicating in four or five days the craving, or even the desire, for drink. On the first day nothing special is done, but on the second and subsequent days an emetic, nearly always tartar emetic or apomorphia, both of which are tasteless and very soluble, is placed in the alcohol, or given hypodermically, in such gradually-increasing dosage that the alcohol excites ever more nausea and repugnance till, if persisted in, such severe vomiting results that it has perforce to be declined. The proof of the pudding is in the eating, and the patient, knowing nothing of the actual cause of his vomiting, ascribes it to the super-excellence of the treatment and is duly impressed. But, and this is a masterpiece of foresight, when, after his six weeks or so of residence, the patient is sent home, he is put in touch with a local club, where he meets old patients, all talking about the wonders of the cure and burning with enthusiasm, a band of allies

HYSTERIA

and heroes whom it would be shameful to desert; in short, the stimuli of enthusiasm and success are behind the cured one, while the special disgrace of black treachery holds in front of him a restraining hand. By a similar wise plan the Salvation Army secures its potential backsliders from dropping back into the mire.

With the Alcoholic as with the Hysteric, any sudden shock may cure even permanently. Many years ago I knew an Aberdeen bailie who, after years of addiction to the wine of his country, was so intensely shocked one morning, after copious libations to Bacchus, on finding that he had broken all his windows and lost a valuable watch and other things overnight, that he gave way to a copious flood of tears and never again—and he lived for many years—took alcohol in any shape or form. While two years later a lady who had been bedridden for years, and about whose actual state doctors had differed widely, some thinking that she had organic nerve disease, on losing her entire fortune in the failure of the Australian Banks, rose and went straight out to the Antipodes to a brother, whose active and

competent housekeeper she became henceforward.

But, in general, the rule holds good that in Hysteria, in order to really cure it, to make the sufferer normal in her response to the normal stimuli of everyday life, you must not lose sight of the patient till you have seen her comfortable, contented and happy in suitable surroundings.

And since your first and only duty is to cure your patient, *cito, tuto et jucunde*, according to the old formula, you must not despise faith-healing and similar measures. Nor must you be disturbed for one moment by thoughtless remarks about the absurdity and fraud of miracles, and the dishonesty of those who make use of them or venture to defend them in modern days. Such remarks show a confusion of thought, and you may be simultaneously on the side of science and that of the angels if you desire it, for science tells us that it is our minds that interpret, if indeed they do not make, the external world. Let the blood but contain a novel ingredient so slight as to escape even the microscopist and the chemist, and, lo and behold! sight, sound,

HYSTERIA

touch, taste and smell may all so alter that a garden of Eden or a Gehenna may come into existence. A poison, you say. There are no poisons as such in nature, and the new ingredient need not even be deleterious; it only need be *different* to the usual run of blood ingredients to produce a miracle in the partaker; and if it were so widely diffused that all absorbed it, then the world would be changed for all of us, and with it even our present conceptions of time and space, nay, even the simplest facts of arithmetic might cease to hold good. We have abundant proof of this in the taker of Indian hemp, of opium, of cocaine and of other drugs, or even of alcohol in excess, and in the wide divergence of views in different nations and at different epochs in history. A Chinaman in New Zealand once told me that he had his heaven with him and exhibited a chunk of crude opium. You have only to imagine a race of men without the sense of sight to whom a man with vision would be one with miraculous faculties, since no one else could conceive of the possibility of sight. Is one single historical fact better sustained than the common existence of dragons

formerly in Europe? Where are they? Our ancestors must have been great liars, a very uncharitable thought, or very credulous, scarcely possible considering that grants of land even in England were made for killing the monsters and much proof would be exacted ere such a reward were given. It is after all but an extension of the moral of the primrose by the river's brim: to one it is nothing more, to another it represents a different world and train of thought. The lesson to be learnt is that there are many mental faculties possible, of which the ordinary man cannot conceive; though of course this should not lead us to accept the reality of wonders without the closest scrutiny of which we are capable.

But I have digressed shamelessly and must pass on.

(5) *Medicinal, electro-therapeutic and mechanical agents.* I have never seen a case of Hysteria cured by any of the above agents, though urgent symptoms have been arrested. The rules I would lay down regarding them are as follows: In the beginning of a treatment, if you have assured yourself that it is within your

HYSTERIA

power to cure the patient by the mental means I have already enumerated, never use any of these agents unless it be with the well-understood reservation that they are recommended only as palliatives and do not enter into your scheme of cure. Otherwise, when they have failed you, as they are sure to do, you will be credited with having shot your best bolt, and any line of treatment you may subsequently adopt will be regarded as in the nature of an afterthought.

In chronic cases in which, for some sufficient reason, you have decided that a radical cure is impossible, drugs and electricity alone are left to you, and then the best possible must be done with them. As in the case of Neurasthenia, tonics in Hysteria almost invariably do harm, if they have any action at all, by increasing the already over-stimulated and hyperactive nervous energy. Therefore those of the nature of strychnia, nux vomica, caffeine and phosphorus are absolutely taboo. If a blood examination shows the presence of anæmia, a mild form of iron may be used, and it is best in that case to combine

it with arsenic. The latter drug, indeed, alone of all the tonics, is ever of real value. It is not stimulating, and it has the effect, if given in very small doses and continuously for months, of improving the physical condition. Bromides are often of service, and if the patient has any objection to the salts of bromide in common use, I order bromide of gold in doses of $\frac{1}{8}$ to $\frac{1}{12}$th grain in pill form, or hydrobromic acid with syrup of lemons. Orange-flower water, greatly in repute in France, may also be given. No hypnotic should ever be ordered unless great care is taken that it cannot be repeated without the doctor's sanction, for hysterical persons are absolutely reckless in their use of drugs, and often so careless about the amount ordered that danger is never far away if several doses of any hypnotic drug are at their command.

Most habitual morphino-maniacs and cocaine fiends have started, as hysterical patients to whom, incautiously, morphia, opium or cocaine has been administered by a doctor or taken in some patent medicine.

Chlorodyne is a great offender in this connection, as are some of the preparations

HYSTERIA

of heroin on the market, and coca wine. And the fact remains that opium and its derivatives, alone of all drugs, seem to have the actual power of curing Hysteria in many cases but at the expense of a far worse disease, the opium habit. That drug stimulates the Ego in a direct way, and amongst its many other drawbacks, converts its victims into the most terrible of egoistic bores. Twenty years ago a lady, whose "dollop," as she styled it, varied from 100 to 150 grains of extract of opium a day, was a source of real terror when she came to consult me. She would wait to see me till she was the last of all the patients, and then, calculating my lunch or dinner hour, beg for all the intermediate time. On the temptation of a conditional promise of marriage from a gentleman to whom she was attached, and who knew of her weakness, she made heroic efforts to conquer the drug, and eventually reduced it to a trivial dose, which she never exceeded. Her previous history is too instructive to omit. As a girl of eighteen she took to her bed, and at twenty-four had both ovaries removed as a means of cure, but obtained no

relief whatever. One day a local doctor happened to call, and promising to cure her, ordered one grain of extract of opium every twelve hours. The first dose removed all her symptoms, a result by no means uncommon. The moral is, never give the drug in Hysteria. Cocaine is nearly equal in efficacy, but far and away more dangerous and terrible in its ultimate effects. The habit, common a few years ago, of taking coca wine often produced hysterical symptoms when the wine was discontinued, and I have been more than once, in former days, puzzled by a sudden and severe attack of Hysteria developing without any discoverable cause in one who had been taking it. One gentleman, who had a bad attack with general tremor, told me that he had been in the habit for some weeks of taking as much as a whole bottle of the wine each evening, feeling " like a god " afterwards. He had no idea that he had been doing a very foolish thing; in fact the wine had been recommended to him as the best remedy for the weakness that follows on influenza.

Laxatives and purgatives should be

HYSTERIA

avoided in all diseases as they gravely derange the ordered muscular action of the intestinal walls, and there is reason to think that their too frequent use is responsible for much of the appendicitis that is now seen. The covered 4lb. or 6lb. cannon ball, allowed to roll its way back and forwards over the surface of the abdomen for about five minutes every morning before rising, is the best remedy for constipation.

Unfortunately in Hysteria we cannot avail ourselves of the " Infallible," that medicine of such marvellous (mental) power in Neurasthenia; for one of the most striking features in which the two disorders differ is in the attitude of the patients towards drugs, which are loved by the Hysteric and dreaded by the Neurasthenic.

Résumé. The cure of Hysteria depends in general on the personality of the doctor, on his knowledge, firmness, judicious sympathy, and above all on the confidence he inspires. Other mental forms of treatment are of occasional service, but drugs should be avoided, and electric treatment used only as a form of " passive exercise " in chronic " bed cases," to maintain the nutrition of

the muscles and nerves and the circulation of the blood.

Disorders mistaken for Neurasthenia and Hysteria

Lying outside my definitions of Neurasthenia and Hysteria there is a state of mental collapse that both in men and women may follow on want of sleep, on prolonged anxiety, and on any protracted struggle against adverse condition; and which is marked by insomnia, irritability, restlessness, depression, inability to make up one's mind in any important matter or to act with decision.

That is *Nervous Breakdown*, and I dealt with it several years ago in a book called *Depression*, for that state is always one of its leading symptoms. Its underlying cause is simple exhaustion of the nervous mechanism and a consequent temporary arrest of the mental faculties, a natural protest by the body against gross misuse and an urgent demand for rest, and sleep. It is to be met at once by absolute rest, and recovery is often aided by the administration of a few doses of bromide of ammonium,

HYSTERIA

which calms the mind and thus permits of natural sleep. After good sleep has been procured, and the patient is restored to fair comfort, it is well to advise him, after first putting his business affairs into order, to take a holiday at some resort where golf, or other suitable diversions, can be enjoyed. Unless there be some special indication to the contrary, he should not be pursued by doctors or by physic, lest his sensitive mind be turned to thoughs of self and Neurasthenia be brought on. If there be cause to suspect any tendency that way it is well to give him an "Infallible" as a stand-by. He must be steered clear of nursing-homes, or of boarding-houses where the conversation chiefly turns on disease, for this variety of Nervous Breakdown is chiefly of importance because it is frequently, if not judiciously treated, the first step on the road to Neurasthenia.

Hypochondriasis, which is often carelessly used as an alternative name for Neurasthenia, should be restricted to its real place, that of a term to connote a well-known variety of Insanity in which *delusions* as to the bodily state exist. It presents a

specious likeness to some kinds of Neurasthenia, while really it is a variety of Melancholia, *i.e.*, of Insanity. It is of great interest to students of Psychology, because the mental condition which it represents is dependent on organic change in some one or more of the abdominal organs, and thus furnishes us with evidence of a statement which I have made elsewhere; that *every cell in the human body probably contributes to mind*, and may be potentially conscious under certain abnormal conditions, even such as under the usual conditions of life contribute to automatic mind, *i.e.*, to the reflex functions, chiefly or solely. One cannot, of course, in the present state of our knowledge be dogmatic on this point, though it has always seemed to me that researches into the causation of some forms of Epilepsy, and most varieties of Melancholia, tend more and more to support my hypothesis. The present fashionable idea in medicine is that the connection between diseased bodily cells and the conscious brain is viâ the blood, and the result of a toxæmia; but if this were so it should be within the powers of science to demonstrate

HYSTERIA

the presence of toxic material in the blood in Epilepsy and in such of the Insanities as have no cerebral morbid anatomy.

The hypochondriac, unlike the Neurasthenic, rests in a delusion. It is a fact to him and he will not bandy words about it. He is not only insensible to, but intolerant of, any argument. "I've got to put up with it and I ought to know all about it," is his pet phrase. His face and manner too are characteristic; for he looks ill, has a set expression and a furtive manner; he is suspicious of everyone, and you never get to really know him; whereas the Neurasthenic is only too willing to unburden his very soul before you, and is anxious that not one single of his many symptoms shall be left out of the reckoning.

But the essential difference between Hypochondriasis and Neurasthenia is that the former is a grave mental disease, rarely recovered from; the victim of which may be fitly compared to a ship in which the cargo has shifted and which has a permanent and dangerous list even in calm weather; whilst the latter is a mere group of symptoms which arise in a *normal* individual when the

surrounding conditions are abnormal; and the sufferer from it is like a well-found ship in a gale, the rolling and tossing of which are but oscillations round a centre of gravity, and essential to its safety under those conditions, and which will, when the storm has abated, again sail calmly over the sea, carrying little or but slight trace of the terrible commotion through which it has passed.

The Neuroses of the Alcoholic and of drug *habitués* may sometimes simulate Neurasthenia, especially those that are seen when the victim is making an effort to overcome his weakness, but the history of the case, the absence of any " bogy," together with the extreme prostration and listlessness, soon undeceive an observer. This stage of distress in recovery from great alcoholic excess and drug-taking is one not devoid of danger to life, and the mental depression that accompanies it is not only extreme but liable to sudden exacerbations. I say this because it is a popular delusion that Alcoholics and others, by some act of will, can at once reform, and may expect a rapid improvement in their health by so doing. Such is not the case. If the person has become more

HYSTERIA

or less immune to the substance taken, he may enjoy good and even excellent health whilst indulging himself, and must be warned not to be daunted by the months of ill-health that will succeed to his most commendable resolve to free himself of the tyranny.

The above are the disorders that are occasionally brought to me, even by doctors, as cases of Neurasthenia, and the absurd nomenclature of use in medicine is alone responsible for the confusion. By reason of such misunderstanding, I have found myself compelled to refer to them, though they are quite outside the scope of this book and are not breaches of the principles laid down in my Preface and earlier chapters.

CHAPTER IX

MENTAL FORMULÆ

MIND as a term is undefinable and as a process unthinkable. We simply have to accept it, to assume it, and to make the best effort possible to classify its various powers, always keeping in mind that, though its control centres have their *pieds-à-terre* in the brain, yet each cell of the body adds its quota to the product, and, like the private soldier, makes the army of which the direction is in the hands of comparatively few specially-trained men. Its division, made solely for convenience, into conscious, subconscious and unconscious, is even artificial, since there is a free communication between them all. How then can we assign values; and how are the values to be expressed; and how are we to allow for the essential fluidity of mind and for the consequent perpetual shifting of our values? The problem is insoluble.

MENTAL FORMULÆ

Yet it would be useful and instructive to have some plan, however elementary, to enable us to visualize the way in which, as far as we can judge, the mind works when it is "made up," when its balance has been effected; and therefore I venture to make the attempt.

The environment supplies the energy with which we have to do mental work, and this energy is utilized in two ways; it is either *inhibited* and stored as memory or reserve energy of some kind; or *exhibited* and used in the production of thought and new combinations of ideas, or in action of some kind.

What decides the relative proportion of this division? The Will, but if you ask me further to give the origin of this faculty of Will I can only answer, that it must be viewed either as a direct emanation from a higher mind (the Heilige Geist), or as the outcome of the varying forces, exerted by the general opinion of the day (the Zeitgeist or Weltgeist), upon the mind of each one of us; the pressure and direction of public opinion, as the newspapers would phrase it. That the individual Will can also, under certain conditions and to a limited extent,

be directly and potently affected by another mind we see in hypnotism, in spiritualism, and in the result of a stern word of command on wavering troops in battle; but we also seem ourselves to possess in some undefinable way a power of control and direction over it.

We will assume that the three usual divisions of the mind are valid ones, for both observation and experiment incline us to the acceptance of this as a general truth; and selecting quite arbitrarily the number 100 as the sum of mental energy in the mind, we will try and assign such a due proportion of it to each division as we should expect to find in a normal masculine and a normal feminine mind; and then we shall be able to understand why the conditions underlying Neurasthenia and Hysteria inevitably lead to the increase of activities in certain directions and to their necessary decrease in others; in short, we shall thus see why the Neurasthenic *must reason* and why the Hysteric *must* show explosive activities in one direction and a more or less complete loss of activity in others.

MENTAL FORMULÆ

Normal Average Masculine Type of Mind

Determined by effect of *will* and *habit*

Environment	Total Amount	Distribution	
		Inhibited	Exhibited
Conscious Portion			
A. Ideas relating to self	30	15	15
B. Ideas relating to others	15	10	5
C. Sensations (impressions)	15	5	10
Subconscious Portion			
D. Instincts	10	8	2
E. Impulses and intuitions	10	8	2
Unconscious Portion			
G. Reflex muscular and secretory impulses	20	8	12
	100	54	46

The above is taken as representative of the ordinary average distribution of energy as determined by the effect of will and by habit. Habit is not a separate faculty, but merely a line of least resistance, the outcome of frequent use in one direction.

In Neurasthenia

Environment	Total Amount	Distribution	
		Inhibited	Exhibited
Conscious Portion			
A (+)	40	10	30
B (−)	5	3	2
C (− in general impressions; + in such as relate to self)	15	5	10

Environment	Total Amount	Distribution	
		Inhibited	Exhibited
Subconscious Portion			
D	10	8	2
E	10	8	2
Unconscious Portion			
G	20	8	12
	100	42	58

The normal proportions are seen to be upset, and 42% of the activities of the conscious mind is exhibited as reasoning activity in place of the normal 30%, while only 15% instead of 30% is stored as memory or diverted into other channels. It is necessary, moreover, to remember that the will power is presumably weakened by the increase of pressure on it at A, and, since the mind is exceedingly fluid, or, to use a better term, elastic, unduly increased in resistance elsewhere. In short, endless disturbance of mental energy is apparently possible, but in the masculine mind the conscious division is so predominant in power that the greatest variation from the normal will be seen there, and this masks the other and minor disturbances which are always present in Neurasthenia if looked for. The great excess in activity of the

MENTAL FORMULÆ

reasoning power is so outstanding a feature in Neurasthenia that the casual observer fails to remark such phenomena as dilatation and sluggishness of the pupils, increased activity of the reflexes, distaste for muscular exertion, partial loss of control over memory (not loss of memory), etc. etc., which one or all, with many others, accompany the disorder.

We now pass to the picture of the feminine mind, viewed first as it is in the normal state, and then as we should expect to see it when in functional disarray.

NORMAL AVERAGE FEMININE TYPE OF MIND

Determined by effect of *will* and *habit*

Environment	Total Amount	Distribution	
		Inhibited	Exhibited
Conscious Portion			
A. Ideas relating to self	20	10	10
B. Ideas relating to others	5	2	3
C. Sensations (impressions)	10	5	5
Subconscious Portion			
D. Instincts	30	25 } restrained by convention	5
E. Impulses and intuitions	15	10 }	5
Unconscious Portion			
G. Reflex muscular and secretory impulsions	20	8	12
	100	55	45

There is here noticeable a tension in the

subconscious portion, a division in which the repressive effects of the Zeitgeist, which is largely the product of the masculine mind as expressed in society, and above all in the press and literature of the day, is evident as a check. The relative proportions of the inhibited and exhibited amounts is thus kept back *under ordinary conditions of life* so as nearly to be identical with that seen in the masculine type of mind.

The reader will also note in the above formula that a larger proportion of the total output of mental energy is assigned to the instincts and impulses of the subconscious mind, and a smaller amount to the conscious mind, than in the masculine mind type. I think that he will agree with me that such a proportionate allowance is in accordance with general experience.

In Hysteria

Environment	Total Amount	Distribution	
		Inhibited	Exhibited
Conscious Portion			
A (+)	27	5	22
B (−)	3	3	0
C (− in such as relate to others; + in such as relate to self) . .	5	1	4

Environment	Total Amount	Distribution	
		Inhibited	Exhibited
Subconscious Portion			
D.	30	10	20
E.	15	1	14
Unconscious Portion			
G.	20	8	12
	100	28	72

The barrier made by subservience to predominant *masculine* popular opinion has gone, broken down as one of the consequences of the disorganization of the formula of health which has arisen largely from an over-development of the self idea, represented by A, and the consequent disturbances of proportionate output.

Again I must ask the reader to remember that these formulæ have no pretence whatever to any exactitude and are introduced only to show graphically, 1st, The general effect of environment; 2nd, The difference in mental constitution between the masculine and feminine minds; 3rd, The disturbance that must ensue chiefly as the result of isolation, of an over-development of self, as a factor in the environment; 4th, The place of will in determining the proportion

in which the mental output of each portion shall be allotted, what part of it shall be stored and what part be expended in mental or physical activities. The part arrested and stored representing the fund of reserve energy always present in the brain and mind. What no formula can represent is the ever-varying power and direction of the will, and the influence of this, and of the environment, in increasing activities in certain directions and paralysing them in others.

What it is desired to teach is that, by studying the environment throughout life, and by training the will, especially in early life, we may avoid, unless possibly much predisposed thereto, the mental and physical troubles that follow on a neglect of those all-important indications.

To forestall, I hope, all criticism I beg the reader to regard the above objects as a valid excuse for presenting him with such elementary formulæ. With the assistance of a friend I some time ago endeavoured to construct more pretentious ones on a wider basis and with the values represented mathematically in considerable detail, but

MENTAL FORMULÆ

the result, though interesting, was even still devoid of any scientific accuracy, while it became so perplexing as to render it unintelligible to any but the mathematical mind and would have been quite out of place in such a book as the present one.

INDEX

ALCOHOL, craving, 151, 166
— cure of habit, 151
Ambitions, 65
Anæmia, 157
Analysis of secretions, etc., 60
Animals and a common mind, 92
Arsenic, 158
Atomism, 1

BALANCE, mental, 7, 15, 28, 37
Bashi-Bazouks, 105
Bastian, Dr Charlton, 6
Bogies, see Phobias and Obsessions
— can be foretold, 53
— how generated, 53
— treatment of, 62, 75
— varieties of, 53 et seq.
Brain, divisions of, 114, 119, 123
— pied-à-terre of mind, 82
Bromides, 49, 158
Burton, Robert, 65

CANNON-BALL, 161
Carlyle, 64
Catalepsy, 118
Celt, 25, 102. 104
Charcot, 66
Charity, 100
China tea, 67
Chlorodyne, 158
Christian Science, 134
Church of England, 104
Climacteric, 112
Coca wine, 160
Cocaine, 160
Common sense, 7, 95

Conventions, 133, 173
Courage in hysteria, 131

DEFINITIONS, faulty, 86
Delusions, 52, 163, 165
Depression, 162
Disease, organic, 47
Disseminated sclerosis, 80
Distress, mental, 8, 13, 114
Double personality, 117
Dramatic appeals, 149
Drugs, 69
— abuse of, 158
— habitués, 166

EGO, 5, 31, 91, 97, 132
Electro-therapy, 156, 161
Emergency medicine, 62
Emotions, 126
Energy in Hysteria, 144
— in Neurasthenia, 43
Environment, 10, 169, 171, 173
Epilepsy, 118, 164
Examination of patient, 60

FACTS, 17
Faddists, 45
Faith-healing, 154
Fasting, 118
Feminine mind type, 24 et seq., 81 et seq.
— best type, 83, 96
— effects of, in history, 25
— failures of balance in, 84, 99
— mental formula of, 173
— three main varieties of, 108
Fibroid tumours, 112
Food fads, 68

Food fads in Neurasthenia, 67
Functional disease, a re-equilibration, 37
— and health, 114
Functions of mind, 5

GALEN, 64
General paralysis, 80
Gift of tongues, 122
Grammar of science, 2

HABIT, 171, 173
Health topics, to be avoided, 71
Heart-beat reduced, 31
Heart-to-heart talk, 129
Heilige Geist, 169
Hermit mind, 41
Home Rule, 103
Hypnotism, 66, 149
Hypochondriasis, 19, 163
— not Neurasthenia, 165
Hysteria, 26, 31, 56, 81, 108 et seq.
— causes of, 31
— contrasted with Insanity, 115
— disequilibration, 28, 81, 95
— disorder of entire brain, 87
— major, 109
— suicide in, 33
— symptoms of, 114
— treatment of, 36, 128 et seq.
Hysterical cases, 32, 116, 123, 134, 144, 150

IMPOSTURE in Hysteria, 115, 125, 136
— in Spiritualism, 90
Indian hemp, 118
Infallible medicines, 62, 163
Insanity, 12, 115, 164
— result of toxæmia, 12
Insomnia, cure of, 146
Instincts, 29, 98, 133
— perverted 120
— starved, 108
Intuition, 24
Isolation, effects of, 23, 40, 94

JAMES, William, 1
Jaundice in hysteria, 123

KNOWLEDGE, contrasted with understanding, 4

LIFE, backwaters of, 42
Logic, 18, 22
Lombroso, 93

MALINGERING, 124, 142
Mapped areas of brain, 6
Marriage, 136
Masculine mind, 17 et seq.
— inferiority of, 96
— predominance of, 18, 100
Melancholia, 52, 164
Mental balance, 7, 13, 27
— comfort, 8, 9, 15
— composition, 9
— equation, 119, 168
— exercises, 70
Mind, balance of, 1 et seq.
— conscious, 5, 171, 173
— divisions of, 114, 119, 123
— great divisions of, 17, 24
— insane, 12
— isolation of, 40
— one and indivisible, 2, 168, 171
— organic (reflex), 5, 171, 173
— the generator, 9
— throws out a balance, 8, 10
Misunderstood persons, 132
Monism, 1
Morphia, 76, 158

NEGATIVISM, 44
Nervous breakdown, 162
Nervous debility, 43
Neurasthenia, absence of organic disease in, 47
— a disequilibration, 81
— a functional disorder, 37
— class of mind affected in, 23
— disorders mistaken for, 162
— energy in, 43
— foods in, 67

INDEX

Neurasthenia, examples of, 49, 50, 63, 73, 79
— sexual, 72
— suicide in, 51
— symptoms of, 37 *et seq.*
— treatment of, 44, 59 *et seq.*, 77
Numbers three and seven, 56
Nuns, hysteria rare in, 138

OBSESSIONS, *see* Bogies
— how generated, 11, 53
Opinions, written, 61
Opium, Chinese taker of, 155
— in hysteria, 159
Overwork, 39

PARALLEL, running of a, 45
Pearson, Dr Karl, 2
Phobias, 11, 53
Phosphorus, 49, 157
Physiology, parent of anatomy, 82
Practical views, 101
Protoplasm, synthetic, 3
Psychasthenia, 43
Psychic immorality, 116, 137
Puberty, 112
Purgatives, 160

QUACKS, 73
Quinine, 49, 76

RACES of different mind-type, 18, 25
Reason, 101
Reflex functions disturbed, 84, 121, 173
Responsibility in hysteria, 115

Rest cures, bad, 65, 78, 79
— good in nervous breakdown, 162

SCOTS, Lowland, 18
Sensuality, 74
Sexual congress, 136
— neurasthenia, 72
— physiology, 113
Shock as cure, 153
Spiritualism, 89
Strain and stress, 42
Strychnine, 49, 76, 157
Suffragist movement, 103
Suicide, 33, 51, 52
Sympathetic ganglia, 7
Syphiliphobia, 45

THEORIES as counterbalances, 8, 27, 35, 53
Tobacco, 69
Tonics, 157
Toxæmia, 164
Traumatic hysteria, 142

VEGETARIANISM, 68
Virility, loss of, 73
Vis Medicatrix Naturæ, 38
Vomiting, fæcal, 124

WEIR-MITCHELL system, 139
Will, 169
Women, kind fitted for work, 111
Work, 39, 50, 63, 142
Worry, 39

ZEITGEIST, 134, 169
— defined, 35

EDINBURGH
COLSTONS LIMITED
PRINTERS

A SELECTION OF BOOKS PUBLISHED BY METHUEN AND CO. LTD., LONDON 36 ESSEX STREET W.C.

CONTENTS

	PAGE		PAGE
General Literature	2	Little Quarto Shakespeare	20
Ancient Cities	13	Miniature Library	20
Antiquary's Books	13	New Library of Medicine	21
Arden Shakespeare	14	New Library of Music	21
Classics of Art	14	Oxford Biographies	21
'Complete' Series	15	Four Plays	21
Connoisseur's Library	15	States of Italy	21
Handbooks of English Church History	16	Westminster Commentaries	22
		'Young' Series	22
Handbooks of Theology	16	Shilling Library	22
'Home Life' Series	16	Books for Travellers	23
Illustrated Pocket Library of Plain and Coloured Books	16	Some Books on Art	23
Leaders of Religion	17	Some Books on Italy	24
Library of Devotion	17	Fiction	25
Little Books on Art	18	Two-Shilling Novels	30
Little Galleries	18	Books for Boys and Girls	30
Little Guides	18	Shilling Novels	31
Little Library	19	Sevenpenny Novels	31

JULY 1913

A SELECTION OF

MESSRS. METHUEN'S PUBLICATIONS

IN this Catalogue the order is according to authors. An asterisk denotes that the book is in the press.

Colonial Editions are published of all Messrs. METHUEN's Novels issued at a price above 2s. 6d., and similar editions are published of some works of General Literature. Colonial Editions are only for circulation in the British Colonies and India.

All books marked net are not subject to discount, and cannot be bought at less than the published price. Books not marked net are subject to the discount which the bookseller allows.

Messrs. METHUEN's books are kept in stock by all good booksellers. If there is any difficulty in seeing copies, Messrs. Methuen will be very glad to have early information, and specimen copies of any books will be sent on receipt of the published price *plus* postage for net books, and of the published price for ordinary books.

This Catalogue contains only a selection of the more important books published by Messrs. Methuen. A complete and illustrated catalogue of their publications may be obtained on application.

Andrewes (Lancelot). PRECES PRIVATAE. Translated and edited, with Notes, by F. E. BRIGHTMAN. *Cr. 8vo.* 6s.

Aristotle. THE ETHICS. Edited, with an Introduction and Notes, by JOHN BURNET. *Demy 8vo.* 10s. 6d. net.

Atkinson (C. T.). A HISTORY OF GERMANY, 1715-1815. *Demy 8vo.* 12s. 6d. net.

Atkinson (T. D.). ENGLISH ARCHITECTURE. Illustrated. *Third Edition. Fcap. 8vo.* 3s. 6d. net.
A GLOSSARY OF TERMS USED IN ENGLISH ARCHITECTURE. Illustrated. *Second Edition. Fcap. 8vo.* 3s. 6d. net.
ENGLISH AND WELSH CATHEDRALS. Illustrated. *Demy 8vo.* 10s. 6d. net.

Bain (F. W.). A DIGIT OF THE MOON: A HINDOO LOVE STORY. *Tenth Edition. Fcap. 8vo.* 3s. 6d. net.
THE DESCENT OF THE SUN: A CYCLE OF BIRTH. *Fifth Edition. Fcap. 8vo.* 3s. 6d. net.
A HEIFER OF THE DAWN. *Seventh Edition. Fcap. 8vo.* 2s. 6d. net.
IN THE GREAT GOD'S HAIR. *Fifth Edition. Fcap. 8vo.* 2s. 6d. net.
A DRAUGHT OF THE BLUE. *Fifth Edition. Fcap. 8vo.* 2s. 6d. net.
AN ESSENCE OF THE DUSK. *Third Edition. Fcap. 8vo.* 2s. 6d. net.
AN INCARNATION OF THE SNOW. *Third Edition. Fcap. 8vo.* 3s. 6d. net.
A MINE OF FAULTS. *Second Edition. Fcap. 8vo.* 3s. 6d. net.
THE ASHES OF A GOD. *Second Edition. Fcap. 8vo.* 3s. 6d. net.
BUBBLES OF THE FOAM. *Fcap. 4to.* 5s. net. Also Fcap. 8vo. 3s. 6d. net.

Balfour (Graham). THE LIFE OF ROBERT LOUIS STEVENSON. Illustrated. *Eleventh Edition. In one Volume. Cr. 8vo. Buckram,* 6s. Also Fcap. 8vo. 1s. net.

Baring (Hon. Maurice). A YEAR IN RUSSIA. *Second Edition. Demy 8vo.* 10s. 6d. net.
LANDMARKS IN RUSSIAN LITERATURE. *Second Edition. Cr. 8vo.* 6s. net.
RUSSIAN ESSAYS AND STORIES. *Second Edition. Cr. 8vo.* 5s. net.
THE RUSSIAN PEOPLE. *Demy 8vo.* 15s. net.

GENERAL LITERATURE

Baring-Gould (S.). THE LIFE OF NAPOLEON BONAPARTE. Illustrated. *Second Edition. Royal 8vo. 10s. 6d. net.*
THE TRAGEDY OF THE CÆSARS: A STUDY OF THE CHARACTERS OF THE CÆSARS OF THE JULIAN AND CLAUDIAN HOUSES. Illustrated. *Seventh Edition. Royal 8vo. 10s. 6d. net.*
THE VICAR OF MORWENSTOW. With a Portrait. *Third Edition. Cr. 8vo. 3s. 6d. Also Fcap. 8vo. 1s. net.*
OLD COUNTRY LIFE. Illustrated. *Fifth Edition. Large Cr. 8vo. 6s. Also fcap. 8vo. 1s. net.*
A BOOK OF CORNWALL. Illustrated. *Third Edition. Cr. 8vo. 6s.*
A BOOK OF DARTMOOR. Illustrated. *Second Edition. Cr. 8vo. 6s.*
A BOOK OF DEVON. Illustrated. *Third Edition. Cr. 8vo. 6s.*

Baring-Gould (S.) and Sheppard (H. Fleetwood). A GARLAND OF COUNTRY SONG. English Folk Songs with their Traditional Melodies. *Demy 4to. 6s.*
SONGS OF THE WEST. Folk Songs of Devon and Cornwall. Collected from the Mouths of the People. New and Revised Edition, under the musical editorship of CECIL J. SHARP. *Large Imperial 8vo. 5s. net.*

Barker (E.). THE POLITICAL THOUGHT OF PLATO AND ARISTOTLE. *Demy 8vo. 10s. 6d. net.*

Bastable (C. F.). THE COMMERCE OF NATIONS. *Sixth Edition. Cr. 8vo. 2s. 6d.*

Beckford (Peter). THOUGHTS ON HUNTING. Edited by J. OTHO PAGET. Illustrated. *Third Edition. Demy 8vo. 6s.*

Belloc (H.). PARIS. Illustrated. *Third Edition. Cr. 8vo. 6s.*
HILLS AND THE SEA. *Fourth Edition. Fcap. 8vo. 5s.*
ON NOTHING AND KINDRED SUBJECTS. *Third Edition. Fcap. 8vo. 5s.*
ON EVERYTHING. *Third Edition. Fcap. 8vo. 5s.*
ON SOMETHING. *Second Edition. Fcap. 8vo. 5s.*
FIRST AND LAST. *Second Edition. Fcap. 8vo. 5s.*
THIS AND THAT AND THE OTHER. *Second Edition. Fcap. 8vo. 5s.*
MARIE ANTOINETTE. Illustrated. *Third Edition. Demy 8vo. 15s. net.*
THE PYRENEES. Illustrated. *Second Edition. Demy 8vo. 7s. 6d. net.*

Bennett (W. H.). A PRIMER OF THE BIBLE. *Fifth Edition. Cr. 8vo. 2s. 6d.*

Bennett (W. H.) and Adeney (W. F.). A BIBLICAL INTRODUCTION. With a concise Bibliography. *Sixth Edition. Cr. 8vo. 7s. 6d. Also in Two Volumes. Cr. 8vo. Each 3s. 6d. net.*

Benson (Archbishop). GOD'S BOARD. Communion Addresses. *Second Edition. Fcap. 8vo. 3s. 6d. net.*

*****Berriman (Algernon E.).** AVIATION. Illustrated. *Cr. 8vo. 5s. net.*

Bicknell (Ethel E.). PARIS AND HER TREASURES. Illustrated. *Fcap. 8vo. Round corners. 5s. net.*

Blake (William). ILLUSTRATIONS OF THE BOOK OF JOB. With a General Introduction by LAURENCE BINYON. Illustrated. *Quarto. 21s. net.*

Bloemfontein (Bishop of). ARA CŒLI: AN ESSAY IN MYSTICAL THEOLOGY. *Fifth Edition. Cr. 8vo. 3s. 6d. net.*
FAITH AND EXPERIENCE. *Second Edition. Cr. 8vo. 3s. 6d. net.*

Bowden (E. M.). THE IMITATION OF BUDDHA. Quotations from Buddhist Literature for each Day in the Year. *Sixth Edition. Cr. 16mo. 2s. 6d.*

Brabant (F. G.). RAMBLES IN SUSSEX. Illustrated. *Cr. 8vo. 6s.*

Bradley (A. G.). ROUND ABOUT WILTSHIRE. Illustrated. *Second Edition. Cr. 8vo. 6s.*
THE ROMANCE OF NORTHUMBERLAND. Illustrated. *Third Edition. Demy 8vo. 7s. 6d. net.*

Braid (James). ADVANCED GOLF. Illustrated. *Seventh Edition. Demy 8vo. 10s. 6d. net.*

Brodrick (Mary) and Morton (A. Anderson). A CONCISE DICTIONARY OF EGYPTIAN ARCHÆOLOGY. A Handbook for Students and Travellers. Illustrated. *Cr. 8vo. 3s. 6d.*

Browning (Robert). PARACELSUS. Edited with an Introduction, Notes, and Bibliography by MARGARET L. LEE and KATHARINE B. LOCOCK. *Fcap. 8vo. 3s. 6d. net.*

Buckton (A. M.). EAGER HEART: A CHRISTMAS MYSTERY-PLAY. *Eleventh Edition. Cr. 8vo. 1s. net.*

Bull (Paul). GOD AND OUR SOLDIERS. *Second Edition. Cr. 8vo. 6s.*

Burns (Robert). THE POEMS AND SONGS. Edited by ANDREW LANG and W. A. CRAIGIE. With Portrait. *Third Edition. Wide Demy 8vo. 6s.*

METHUEN AND COMPANY LIMITED

Calman (W. T.). THE LIFE OF CRUSTACEA. Illustrated. *Cr. 8vo. 6s.*

Carlyle (Thomas). THE FRENCH REVOLUTION. Edited by C. R. L. FLETCHER. *Three Volumes. Cr. 8vo. 18s.*
THE LETTERS AND SPEECHES OF OLIVER CROMWELL. With an Introduction by C. H. FIRTH, and Notes and Appendices by S. C. LOMAS. *Three Volumes. Demy 8vo. 18s. net.*

Celano (Brother Thomas of). THE LIVES OF S. FRANCIS OF ASSISI. Translated by A. G. FERRERS HOWELL. With a Frontispiece. *Cr. 8vo. 5s. net.*

Chambers (Mrs. Lambert). LAWN TENNIS FOR LADIES. Illustrated. *Second Edition. Cr. 8vo. 2s. 6d. net.*

Chesser (Elizabeth Sloan). PERFECT HEALTH FOR WOMEN AND CHILDREN. *Cr. 8vo. 3s. 6d. net.*

Chesterfield (Lord). THE LETTERS OF THE EARL OF CHESTERFIELD TO HIS SON. Edited, with an Introduction by C. STRACHEY, and Notes by A. CALTHROP. *Two Volumes. Cr. 8vo. 12s.*

Chesterton (G. K.). CHARLES DICKENS. With two Portraits in Photogravure. *Eighth Edition. Cr. 8vo. 6s.*
ALL THINGS CONSIDERED. *Seventh Edition. Fcap. 8vo. 5s.*
TREMENDOUS TRIFLES. *Fifth Edition. Fcap. 8vo. 5s.*
ALARMS AND DISCURSIONS. *Second Edition. Fcap. 8vo. 5s.*
THE BALLAD OF THE WHITE HORSE. *Fourth Edition. Fcap. 8vo. 5s.*
A MISCELLANY OF MEN. *Second Edition. Fcap. 8vo. 5s.*

Clausen (George). SIX LECTURES ON PAINTING. Illustrated. *Third Edition. Large Post 8vo. 3s. 6d. net.*
AIMS AND IDEALS IN ART. Eight Lectures delivered to the Students of the Royal Academy of Arts. Illustrated. *Second Edition. Large Post 8vo. 5s. net.*

Clutton-Brock (A.). SHELLEY: THE MAN AND THE POET. Illustrated. *Demy 8vo. 7s. 6d. net.*

Cobb (W. F.). THE BOOK OF PSALMS. With an Introduction and Notes. *Demy 8vo. 10s. 6d. net.*

Conrad (Joseph). THE MIRROR OF THE SEA: Memories and Impressions. *Fourth Edition. Fcap. 8vo. 5s.*

Coolidge (W. A. B.). THE ALPS: IN NATURE AND HISTORY. Illustrated. *Demy 8vo. 7s. 6d. net.*

Correvon (H.). ALPINE FLORA. Translated and enlarged by E. W. CLAYFORTH. Illustrated. *Square Demy 8vo. 16s. net.*

Coulton (G. G.). CHAUCER AND HIS ENGLAND. Illustrated. *Second Edition. Demy 8vo. 10s. 6d. net.*

Cowper (William). THE POEMS. Edited, with an Introduction and Notes, by J. C. BAILEY. Illustrated. *Demy 8vo. 10s. 6d. net.*

Cox (J. C.). RAMBLES IN SURREY. Illustrated. *Second Edition. Cr. 8vo. 6s.*
RAMBLES IN KENT. Illustrated. *Cr. 8vo. 6s.*

Crowley (H. Ralph). THE HYGIENE OF SCHOOL LIFE. Illustrated. *Cr. 8vo. 3s. 6d. net.*

Davis (H. W. C.). ENGLAND UNDER THE NORMANS AND ANGEVINS: 1066-1272. *Third Edition. Demy 8vo. 10s. 6d. net.*

Dawbarn (Charles). FRANCE AND THE FRENCH. Illustrated. *Demy 8vo. 10s. 6d. net.*

Dearmer (Mabel). A CHILD'S LIFE OF CHRIST. Illustrated. *Large Cr. 8vo. 6s.*

Deffand (Madame du). LETTRES DE LA MARQUISE DU DEFFAND À HORACE WALPOLE. Edited, with Introduction, Notes, and Index, by Mrs. PAGET TOYNBEE. *In Three Volumes. Demy 8vo. £3 3s. net.*

Dickinson (G. L.). THE GREEK VIEW OF LIFE. *Eighth Edition. Cr. 8vo. 2s. 6d. net.*

Ditchfield (P. H.). THE PARISH CLERK. *Fcap. 8vo. 1s. net.*
THE OLD-TIME PARSON. Illustrated. *Second Edition. Demy 8vo. 7s. 6d. net.*
THE OLD ENGLISH COUNTRY SQUIRE. Illustrated. *Demy 8vo. 10s. 6d. net.*

Ditchfield (P. H.) and Roe (Fred). VANISHING ENGLAND. The Book by P. H. DITCHFIELD. Illustrated by FRED ROE. *Second Edition. Wide Demy 8vo. 15s. net.*

Douglas (Hugh A.). VENICE ON FOOT. With the Itinerary of the Grand Canal. Illustrated. *Second Edition. Round corners. Fcap. 8vo. 5s. net.*
VENICE AND HER TREASURES. Illustrated. *Round corners. Fcap. 8vo. 5s. net.*

GENERAL LITERATURE

Dowden (J.). FURTHER STUDIES IN THE PRAYER BOOK. *Cr. 8vo.* 6s.

Driver (S. R.). SERMONS ON SUBJECTS CONNECTED WITH THE OLD TESTAMENT. *Cr. 8vo.* 6s.

Dumas (Alexandre). THE CRIMES OF THE BORGIAS AND OTHERS. With an Introduction by R. S. GARNETT. Illustrated. *Second Edition. Cr. 8vo.* 6s.

THE CRIMES OF URBAIN GRANDIER AND OTHERS. Illustrated. *Cr. 8vo.* 6s.

THE CRIMES OF THE MARQUISE DE BRINVILLIERS AND OTHERS. Illustrated. *Cr. 8vo.* 6s.

THE CRIMES OF ALI PASHA AND OTHERS. Illustrated. *Cr. 8vo.* 6s.

MY PETS. Newly translated by A. R. ALLINSON. Illustrated. *Cr. 8vo.* 6s.

Duncan (F. M.). OUR INSECT FRIENDS AND FOES. Illustrated. *Cr. 8vo.* 6s.

Dunn-Pattison (R. P.). NAPOLEON'S MARSHALS. Illustrated. *Second Edition. Demy 8vo.* 12s. 6d. net.

THE BLACK PRINCE. Illustrated. *Second Edition. Demy 8vo.* 7s. 6d. net.

Durham (The Earl of). THE REPORT ON CANADA. With an Introductory Note. *Demy 8vo.* 4s. 6d. net.

Dutt (W. A.). THE NORFOLK BROADS. Illustrated. *Second Edition. Cr. 8vo.* 6s.

Egerton (H. E.). A SHORT HISTORY OF BRITISH COLONIAL POLICY. *Third Edition. Demy 8vo.* 7s. 6d. net.

Evans (Herbert A.). CASTLES OF ENGLAND AND WALES. Illustrated. *Demy 8vo.* 12s. 6d. net.

Exeter (Bishop of). REGNUM DEI. (The Bampton Lectures of 1901.) *A Cheaper Edition. Demy 8vo.* 7s. 6d. net.

Ewald (Carl). MY LITTLE BOY. Translated by ALEXANDER TEIXEIRA DE MATTOS. Illustrated. *Fcap. 8vo.* 5s.

Fairbrother (W. H.). THE PHILOSOPHY OF T. H. GREEN. *Second Edition. Cr. 8vo.* 3s. 6d.

ffoulkes (Charles). THE ARMOURER AND HIS CRAFT. Illustrated. *Royal 4to.* £2 2s. net.

Firth (C. H.). CROMWELL'S ARMY. A History of the English Soldier during the Civil Wars, the Commonwealth, and the Protectorate. Illustrated. *Second Edition. Cr. 8vo.* 6s.

Fisher (H. A. L.). THE REPUBLICAN TRADITION IN EUROPE. *Cr. 8vo.* 6s. net.

FitzGerald (Edward). THE RUBAI'YÁT OF OMAR KHAYYÁM. Printed from the Fifth and last Edition. With a Commentary by H. M. BATSON, and a Biographical Introduction by E. D. ROSS. *Cr. 8vo.* 6s.

Flux (A. W.). ECONOMIC PRINCIPLES. *Demy 8vo.* 7s. 6d. net.

Fraser (E.). THE SOLDIERS WHOM WELLINGTON LED. Deeds of Daring, Chivalry, and Renown. Illustrated. *Cr. 8vo.* 5s. net.

Fraser (J. F.). ROUND THE WORLD ON A WHEEL. Illustrated. *Fifth Edition. Cr. 8vo.* 6s.

Galton (Sir Francis). MEMORIES OF MY LIFE. Illustrated. *Third Edition. Demy 8vo.* 10s. 6d. net.

Gibbins (H. de B.). INDUSTRY IN ENGLAND: HISTORICAL OUTLINES. With Maps and Plans. *Seventh Edition, Revised. Demy 8vo.* 10s. 6d.

THE INDUSTRIAL HISTORY OF ENGLAND. With 5 Maps and a Plan. *Nineteenth Edition. Cr. 8vo.* 3s.

ENGLISH SOCIAL REFORMERS. *Second Edition. Cr. 8vo.* 2s. 6d.

Gibbon (Edward). THE MEMOIRS OF THE LIFE OF EDWARD GIBBON. Edited by G. BIRKBECK HILL. *Cr. 8vo.* 6s.

THE DECLINE AND FALL OF THE ROMAN EMPIRE. Edited, with Notes, Appendices, and Maps, by J. B. BURY, Illustrated. *In Seven Volumes. Demy 8vo.* Each 10s. 6d. net. *Also in Seven Volumes. Cr. 8vo.* 6s. each.

Glover (T. R.). THE CONFLICT OF RELIGIONS IN THE EARLY ROMAN EMPIRE. *Fourth Edition. Demy 8vo.* 7s. 6d. net.

VIRGIL. *Second Edition. Demy 8vo.* 7s. 6d. net.

*THE CHRISTIAN TRADITION AND ITS VERIFICATION. (The Angus Lecture for 1912.) *Cr. 8vo.* 3s. 6d. net.

Godley (A. D.). LYRA FRIVOLA. *Fourth Edition. Fcap. 8vo.* 2s. 6d.
VERSES TO ORDER. *Second Edition. Fcap. 8vo.* 2s. 6d.
SECOND STRINGS. *Fcap. 8vo.* 2s. 6d.

Gostling (Frances M.). THE BRETONS AT HOME. Illustrated. *Second Edition. Cr. 8vo.* 6s.
AUVERGNE AND ITS PEOPLE. Illustrated. *Demy 8vo.* 10s. 6d. net.

Gray (Arthur). CAMBRIDGE. Illustrated. *Demy 8vo.* 7s. 6d. net.

Grahame (Kenneth). THE WIND IN THE WILLOWS. Illustrated. *Seventh Edition. Cr. 8vo.* 6s.

Granger (Frank). HISTORICAL SOCIOLOGY: A TEXT-BOOK OF POLITICS. *Cr. 8vo.* 3s. 6d. net.

Grew (Edwin Sharpe). THE GROWTH OF A PLANET. Illustrated. *Cr. 8vo.* 6s.

Griffin (W. Hall) and Minchin (H. C.). THE LIFE OF ROBERT BROWNING. Illustrated. *Second Edition. Demy 8vo.* 12s. 6d. net.

Haig (K. G.). HEALTH THROUGH DIET. *Second Edition. Cr. 8vo.* 3s. 6d. net.

Hale (J. R.). FAMOUS SEA FIGHTS: FROM SALAMIS TO TSU-SHIMA. Illustrated. *Second Edition. Cr. 8vo.* 6s. net.

Hall (H. R.). THE ANCIENT HISTORY OF THE NEAR EAST FROM THE EARLIEST TIMES TO THE BATTLE OF SALAMIS. Illustrated. *Demy 8vo.* 15s. net.

Hannay (D.). A SHORT HISTORY OF THE ROYAL NAVY. Vol. I., 1217–1688. Vol. II., 1689–1815. *Demy 8vo.* Each 7s. 6d.

Hare (B.). THE GOLFING SWING. *Third Edition. Fcap. 8vo.* 1s. net.

Harper (Charles G.). THE AUTOCAR ROAD-BOOK. With Maps. *In Four Volumes. Cr. 8vo.* Each 7s. 6d. net.

Vol. I.—SOUTH OF THE THAMES.
Vol. II.—NORTH AND SOUTH WALES AND WEST MIDLANDS.
Vol. III.—EAST ANGLIA AND EAST MIDLANDS.
*Vol. IV.—THE NORTH OF ENGLAND AND SOUTH OF SCOTLAND.

Harris (Frank). THE WOMEN OF SHAKESPEARE. *Demy 8vo.* 7s. 6d. net.

Hassall (Arthur). THE LIFE OF NAPOLEON. Illustrated. *Demy 8vo.* 7s. 6d. net.

Headley (F. W.). DARWINISM AND MODERN SOCIALISM. *Second Edition. Cr. 8vo.* 5s. net.

Henderson (M. Sturge). GEORGE MEREDITH: NOVELIST, POET, REFORMER. With a Portrait. *Second Edition. Cr. 8vo.* 6s.

Henley (W. E.). ENGLISH LYRICS: CHAUCER TO POE. *Second Edition. Cr. 8vo.* 2s. 6d. net.

Hill (George Francis). ONE HUNDRED MASTERPIECES OF SCULPTURE. Illustrated. *Demy 8vo.* 10s. 6d. net.

Hind (C. Lewis). DAYS IN CORNWALL. Illustrated. *Third Edition. Cr. 8vo.* 6s.

Hobhouse (L. T.). THE THEORY OF KNOWLEDGE. *Demy 8vo.* 10s. 6d. net.

Hobson (J. A.). INTERNATIONAL TRADE: AN APPLICATION OF ECONOMIC THEORY. *Cr. 8vo.* 2s. 6d. net.
PROBLEMS OF POVERTY: AN INQUIRY INTO THE INDUSTRIAL CONDITION OF THE POOR. *Eighth Edition. Cr. 8vo.* 2s. 6d.
THE PROBLEM OF THE UNEMPLOYED: AN INQUIRY AND AN ECONOMIC POLICY. *Fifth Edition. Cr. 8vo.* 2s. 6d.
GOLD, PRICES AND WAGES. *Cr. 8vo.* 3s. 6d. net.

Hodgson (Mrs. W.). HOW TO IDENTIFY OLD CHINESE PORCELAIN. Illustrated. *Third Edition. Post 8vo.* 6s.

Holdich (Sir T. H.). THE INDIAN BORDERLAND, 1880–1900. Illustrated. *Second Edition. Demy 8vo.* 10s. 6d. net.

Holdsworth (W. S.). A HISTORY OF ENGLISH LAW. *In Four Volumes. Vols. I., II., III. Demy 8vo.* Each 10s. 6d. net.

Holland (Clive). TYROL AND ITS PEOPLE. Illustrated. *Demy 8vo.* 10s. 6d. net.
THE BELGIANS AT HOME. Illustrated. *Demy 8vo.* 10s. 6d. net.

Horsburgh (E. L. S.). LORENZO THE MAGNIFICENT; AND FLORENCE IN HER GOLDEN AGE. Illustrated. *Second Edition. Demy 8vo.* 15s. net.
WATERLOO: A NARRATIVE AND A CRITICISM. With Plans. *Second Edition. Cr. 8vo.* 5s.

GENERAL LITERATURE

THE LIFE OF SAVONAROLA. Illustrated. *Cr. 8vo. 5s. net.*

Hosie (Alexander). MANCHURIA. Illustrated. *Second Edition. Demy 8vo. 7s. 6d. net.*

Hudson (W. H.). A SHEPHERD'S LIFE: IMPRESSIONS OF THE SOUTH WILTSHIRE DOWNS. Illustrated. *Third Edition. Demy 8vo. 7s. 6d. net.*

Humphreys (John H.). PROPORTIONAL REPRESENTATION. *Cr. 8vo. 5s. net.*

Hutchinson (Horace G.). THE NEW FOREST. Illustrated. *Fourth Edition. Cr. 8vo. 6s.*

Hutton (Edward). THE CITIES OF SPAIN. Illustrated. *Fourth Edition. Cr. 8vo. 6s.*
THE CITIES OF UMBRIA. Illustrated. *Fifth Edition. Cr. 8vo. 6s.*
THE CITIES OF LOMBARDY. Illustrated. *Cr. 8vo. 6s.*
FLORENCE AND NORTHERN TUSCANY WITH GENOA. Illustrated. *Second Edition. Cr. 8vo. 6s.*
SIENA AND SOUTHERN TUSCANY. Illustrated. *Second Edition. Cr. 8vo. 6s.*
VENICE AND VENETIA. Illustrated. *Cr. 8vo. 6s.*
ROME. Illustrated. *Third Edition. Cr. 8vo. 6s.*
COUNTRY WALKS ABOUT FLORENCE. Illustrated. *Second Edition. Fcap. 8vo. 5s. net.*
IN UNKNOWN TUSCANY, With Notes by WILLIAM HEYWOOD. Illustrated. *Second Edition. Demy 8vo. 7s. 6d. net.*
A BOOK OF THE WYE. Illustrated. *Demy 8vo. 7s. 6d. net.*

Ibsen (Henrik). BRAND. A Dramatic Poem, translated by WILLIAM WILSON. *Fourth Edition. Cr. 8vo. 3s. 6d.*

Inge (W. R.). CHRISTIAN MYSTICISM. (The Bampton Lectures of 1899.) *Third Edition. Cr. 8vo. 5s. net.*

Innes (A. D.). A HISTORY OF THE BRITISH IN INDIA. With Maps and Plans. *Cr. 8vo. 6s.*
ENGLAND UNDER THE TUDORS. With Maps. *Third Edition. Demy 8vo. 10s. 6d. net.*

Innes (Mary). SCHOOLS OF PAINTING. Illustrated. *Second Edition. Cr. 8vo. 5s. net.*

Jenks (E.). AN OUTLINE OF ENGLISH LOCAL GOVERNMENT. *Second Edition.* Revised by R. C. K. ENSOR. *Cr. 8vo. 2s. 6d. net.*
A SHORT HISTORY OF ENGLISH LAW: FROM THE EARLIEST TIMES TO THE END OF THE YEAR 1911. *Demy 8vo. 10s. 6d. net.*

Jerningham (Charles Edward). THE MAXIMS OF MARMADUKE. *Second Edition. Cr. 8vo. 5s.*

Jevons (F. B.). PERSONALITY. *Cr. 8vo. 2s. 6d. net.*

Johnston (Sir H. H.). BRITISH CENTRAL AFRICA. Illustrated. *Third Edition. Cr. 4to. 18s. net.*
THE NEGRO IN THE NEW WORLD. Illustrated. *Demy 8vo. 21s. net.*

Julian (Lady) of Norwich. REVELATIONS OF DIVINE LOVE. Edited by GRACE WARRACK. *Fourth Edition. Cr. 8vo. 3s. 6d.*

Keats (John). THE POEMS. Edited, with Introduction and Notes, by E. de SÉLINCOURT. With a Frontispiece in Photogravure. *Third Edition. Demy 8vo. 7s. 6d. net.*

Keble (John). THE CHRISTIAN YEAR. With an Introduction and Notes by W. LOCK. Illustrated. *Third Edition. Fcap. 8vo. 3s. 6d.*

Kempis (Thomas à). THE IMITATION OF CHRIST. From the Latin, with an Introduction by DEAN FARRAR. Illustrated. *Third Edition. Fcap. 8vo. 3s. 6d.*

Kipling (Rudyard). BARRACK-ROOM BALLADS. 114th Thousand. *Thirty-fourth Edition. Cr. 8vo. 6s. Also Fcap. 8vo. Cloth, 4s. 6d. net ; Leather, 5s. net.*
THE SEVEN SEAS. 94th Thousand. *Twenty-first Edition. Cr. 8vo. 6s. Also Fcap. 8vo. Cloth, 4s. 6d. net ; Leather, 5s. net.*
THE FIVE NATIONS. 78th Thousand. *Eleventh Edition. Cr. 8vo. 6s. Also Fcap. 8vo. Cloth, 4s. 6d. net ; Leather, 5s. net.*
DEPARTMENTAL DITTIES. *Twenty-Third Edition. Cr. 8vo. 6s. Also Fcap. 8vo. Cloth, 4s. 6d. net ; Leather, 5s. net.*

Lamb (Charles and Mary). THE COMPLETE WORKS. Edited, with an Introduction and Notes, by E. V. LUCAS. *A New and Revised Edition in Six Volumes.* With Frontispiece. *Fcap. 8vo. 5s. each.*
The volumes are:—
I. MISCELLANEOUS PROSE. II. ELIA AND THE LAST ESSAYS OF ELIA. III. BOOKS FOR CHILDREN. IV. PLAYS AND POEMS. V. and VI. LETTERS.

Lankester (Sir Ray). SCIENCE FROM AN EASY CHAIR. Illustrated. *Seventh Edition. Cr. 8vo. 6s.*

Le Braz (Anatole). THE LAND OF PARDONS. Translated by FRANCES M. GOSTLING. Illustrated. *Fourth Edition. Cr. 8vo. 6s.*

Lee (Gerald Stanley). INSPIRED MILLIONAIRES. *Cr. 8vo. 3s. 6d. net.*
*CROWDS. *Cr. 8vo. 6s.*

Lock (Walter). ST. PAUL, THE MASTER BUILDER. *Third Edition. Cr. 8vo. 3s. 6d.*
THE BIBLE AND CHRISTIAN LIFE. *Cr. 8vo. 6s.*

Lodge (Sir Oliver). THE SUBSTANCE OF FAITH, ALLIED WITH SCIENCE: A CATECHISM FOR PARENTS AND TEACHERS. *Eleventh Edition. Cr. 8vo. 2s. net.*
MAN AND THE UNIVERSE: A STUDY OF THE INFLUENCE OF THE ADVANCE IN SCIENTIFIC KNOWLEDGE UPON OUR UNDERSTANDING OF CHRISTIANITY. *Ninth Edition. Demy 8vo. 5s. net. Also Fcap. 8vo. 1s. net.*
THE SURVIVAL OF MAN: A STUDY IN UNRECOGNISED HUMAN FACULTY. *Fifth Edition. Wide Cr. 8vo. 5s. net.*
REASON AND BELIEF. *Fifth Edition. Cr. 8vo. 3s. 6d. net.*
MODERN PROBLEMS. *Cr. 8vo. 5s. net.*

Lorimer (George Horace). LETTERS FROM A SELF-MADE MERCHANT TO HIS SON. Illustrated. *Twenty-fourth Edition. Cr. 8vo. 3s. 6d. Also Fcap. 8vo. 1s. net.*
OLD GORGON GRAHAM. Illustrated. *Second Edition. Cr. 8vo. 6s. *Also Cr. 8vo. 2s. net.*

Lucas (E. V.). THE LIFE OF CHARLES LAMB. Illustrated. *Fifth Edition. Demy 8vo. 7s. 6d. net.*
A WANDERER IN HOLLAND. Illustrated. *Fourteenth Edition. Cr. 8vo. 6s.*
A WANDERER IN LONDON. Illustrated. *Fourteenth Edition. Cr. 8vo. 6s.*
A WANDERER IN PARIS. Illustrated. *Tenth Edition. Cr. 8vo. 6s. Also Fcap. 8vo. 5s.*
A WANDERER IN FLORENCE. Illustrated. *Fourth Edition. Cr. 8vo. 6s.*
THE OPEN ROAD: A LITTLE BOOK FOR WAYFARERS. *Nineteenth Edition. Fcap. 8vo. 5s. India Paper, 7s. 6d.*
THE FRIENDLY TOWN: A LITTLE BOOK FOR THE URBANE. *Seventh Edition. Fcap. 8vo. 5s.*
FIRESIDE AND SUNSHINE. *Seventh Edition. Fcap 8vo. 5s.*
CHARACTER AND COMEDY. *Sixth Edition. Fcap. 8vo. 5s.*
THE GENTLEST ART: A CHOICE OF LETTERS BY ENTERTAINING HANDS. *Seventh Edition. Fcap. 8vo. 5s.*
THE SECOND POST. *Third Edition. Fcap. 8vo. 5s.*
HER INFINITE VARIETY: A FEMININE PORTRAIT GALLERY. *Sixth Edition. Fcap. 8vo. 5s.*
GOOD COMPANY: A RALLY OF MEN. *Second Edition. Fcap. 8vo. 5s.*
ONE DAY AND ANOTHER. *Fifth Edition. Fcap. 8vo. 5s.*
OLD LAMPS FOR NEW. *Fourth Edition. Fcap. 8vo. 5s.*
LISTENER'S LURE: AN OBLIQUE NARRATION. *Ninth Edition. Fcap. 8vo. 5s.*
OVER BEMERTON'S: AN EASY-GOING CHRONICLE. *Tenth Edition. Fcap. 8vo. 5s.*
MR. INGLESIDE. *Ninth Edition. Fcap. 8vo. 5s.*
THE BRITISH SCHOOL: AN ANECDOTAL GUIDE TO THE BRITISH PAINTERS AND PAINTINGS IN THE NATIONAL GALLERY. *Fcap. 8vo. 2s. 6d. net.*
See also Lamb (Charles).

Lydekker (R.) and Others. REPTILES, AMPHIBIA, FISHES, AND LOWER CHORDATA. Edited by J. C. CUNNINGHAM. Illustrated. *Demy 8vo. 10s. 6d. net.*

Lydekker (R.). THE OX AND ITS KINDRED. Illustrated. *Cr. 8vo. 6s.*

Macaulay (Lord). CRITICAL AND HISTORICAL ESSAYS. Edited by F. C. MONTAGUE. *Three Volumes. Cr. 8vo. 18s.*

McCabe (Joseph). THE DECAY OF THE CHURCH OF ROME. *Third Edition. Demy 8vo. 7s. 6d. net.*
THE EMPRESSES OF ROME. Illustrated. *Demy 8vo. 12s. 6d. net.*

MacCarthy (Desmond) and Russell (Agatha). LADY JOHN RUSSELL: A MEMOIR. Illustrated. *Fourth Edition. Demy 8vo. 10s. 6d. net.*

McCullagh (Francis). THE FALL OF ABD-UL-HAMID. Illustrated. *Demy 8vo. 10s. 6d. net.*

McDougall (William). AN INTRODUCTION TO SOCIAL PSYCHOLOGY. *Sixth Edition. Cr. 8vo. 5s. net.*
BODY AND MIND: A HISTORY AND A DEFENCE OF ANIMISM. *Second Edition Demy 8vo. 10s. 6d. net.*

GENERAL LITERATURE

'Mdlle. Mori' (Author of). ST. CATHERINE OF SIENA AND HER TIMES. Illustrated. *Second Edition. Demy 8vo. 7s. 6d. net.*

Maeterlinck (Maurice). THE BLUE BIRD: A FAIRY PLAY IN SIX ACTS. Translated by ALEXANDER TEIXEIRA DE MATTOS. *Fcap. 8vo. Deckle Edges. 3s. 6d. net. Also Fcap. 8vo. 1s. net.* An Edition, illustrated in colour by F. CAYLEY ROBINSON, is also published. *Cr. 4to. Gilt top. 21s. net.* Of the above book Thirty-three Editions in all have been issued.

MARY MAGDALENE: A PLAY IN THREE ACTS. Translated by ALEXANDER TEIXEIRA DE MATTOS. *Third Edition. Fcap. 8vo. Deckle Edges. 3s. 6d. net. Also Fcap. 8vo. 1s. net.*

DEATH. Translated by ALEXANDER TEIXEIRA DE MATTOS. *Fourth Edition. Fcap. 8vo. 3s. 6d. net.*

Mahaffy (J. P.). A HISTORY OF EGYPT UNDER THE PTOLEMAIC DYNASTY. Illustrated. *Cr. 8vo. 6s.*

Maitland (F. W.). ROMAN CANON LAW IN THE CHURCH OF ENGLAND. *Royal 8vo. 7s. 6d.*

Marett (R. R.). THE THRESHOLD OF RELIGION. *Cr. 8vo. 3s. 6d. net.*

Marriott (Charles). A SPANISH HOLIDAY. Illustrated. *Demy 8vo. 7s. 6d. net.*
THE ROMANCE OF THE RHINE. Illustrated. *Demy 8vo. 10s. 6d. net.*

Marriott (J. A. R.). THE LIFE AND TIMES OF LUCIUS CARY, VISCOUNT FALKLAND. Illustrated. *Second Edition. Demy 8vo. 7s. 6d. net.*
ENGLAND SINCE WATERLOO. *Demy 8vo. 10s. 6d. net.*

Masefield (John). SEA LIFE IN NELSON'S TIME. Illustrated. *Cr. 8vo. 3s. 6d. net.*
A SAILOR'S GARLAND. Selected and Edited. *Second Edition. Cr. 8vo. 3s. 6d. net.*

Masterman (C. F. G.). TENNYSON AS A RELIGIOUS TEACHER. *Second Edition. Cr. 8vo. 6s.*
THE CONDITION OF ENGLAND. *Fourth Edition. Cr. 8vo. 6s. Also Fcap. 8vo. 1s net.*

Mayne (Ethel Colburn). BYRON. Illustrated. *In Two Volumes. Demy 8vo. 21s. net.*

Medley (D. J.). ORIGINAL ILLUSTRATIONS OF ENGLISH CONSTITUTIONAL HISTORY. *Cr. 8vo. 7s. 6d. net.*

Methuen (A. M. S.). ENGLAND'S RUIN: DISCUSSED IN FOURTEEN LETTERS TO A PROTECTIONIST. *Ninth Edition. Cr. 8vo. 3d. net.*

Miles (Eustace). LIFE AFTER LIFE; OR, THE THEORY OF REINCARNATION. *Cr. 8vo. 2s. 6d. net.*
THE POWER OF CONCENTRATION: HOW TO ACQUIRE IT. *Fourth Edition. Cr. 8vo. 3s. 6d. net.*

Millais (J. G.). THE LIFE AND LETTERS OF SIR JOHN EVERETT MILLAIS. Illustrated. *New Edition. Demy 8vo. 7s. 6d. net.*

Milne (J. G.). A HISTORY OF EGYPT UNDER ROMAN RULE. Illustrated. *Cr. 8vo. 6s.*

Moffat (Mary M.). QUEEN LOUISA OF PRUSSIA. Illustrated. *Fourth Edition. Cr. 8vo. 6s.*
MARIA THERESA. Illustrated. *Demy 8vo. 10s. 6d. net.*

Money (L. G. Chiozza). RICHES AND POVERTY. *New and Revised Issue. Cr. 8vo. 1s. net.*
MONEY'S FISCAL DICTIONARY, 1910. *Second Edition. Demy 8vo. 5s. net.*
THINGS THAT MATTER: PAPERS ON SUBJECTS WHICH ARE, OR OUGHT TO BE, UNDER DISCUSSION. *Demy 8vo. 5s. net.*

Montague (C. E.). DRAMATIC VALUES. *Second Edition. Fcap. 8vo. 5s.*

Moorhouse (E. Hallam). NELSON'S LADY HAMILTON. Illustrated. *Third Edition. Demy 8vo. 7s. 6d. net.*

Morgan (C. Lloyd). INSTINCT AND EXPERIENCE. *Second Edition. Cr. 8vo. 5s. net.*

Nevill (Lady Dorothy). MY OWN TIMES. Edited by her Son. *Second Edition. Demy 8vo. 15s. net.*

Norway (A. H.). NAPLES: PAST AND PRESENT. Illustrated. *Fourth Edition. Cr. 8vo. 6s.*

O'Donnell (Elliot). WERWOLVES. *Cr. 8vo. 5s. net.*

Oman (C. W. C.). A HISTORY OF THE ART OF WAR IN THE MIDDLE AGES. Illustrated. *Demy 8vo. 10s. 6d. net.*
ENGLAND BEFORE THE NORMAN CONQUEST. With Maps. *Third Edition, Revised. Demy 8vo. 10s. 6d. net.*

Oxford (M. N.). A HANDBOOK OF NURSING. *Sixth Edition, Revised. Cr. 8vo.* 3s. 6d. *net.*

Pakes (W. C. C.). THE SCIENCE OF HYGIENE. Illustrated. *Second and Cheaper Edition.* Revised by A. T. Nankivell. *Cr. 8vo.* 5s. *net.*

Parker (Eric). A BOOK OF THE ZOO. Illustrated. *Second Edition. Cr. 8vo.* 6s.

Pears (Sir Edwin). TURKEY AND ITS PEOPLE. *Second Edition. Demy 8vo.* 12s. 6d. *net.*

Petrie (W. M. Flinders.) A HISTORY OF EGYPT. Illustrated. *In Six Volumes. Cr. 8vo.* 6s. *each.*

Vol. I. From the Ist to the XVIth Dynasty. *Seventh Edition.*
Vol. II. The XVIIth and XVIIIth Dynasties. *Fourth Edition.*
Vol. III. XIXth to XXXth Dynasties.
Vol. IV. Egypt under the Ptolemaic Dynasty. J. P. Mahaffy.
Vol V. Egypt under Roman Rule. J. G. Milne.
Vol. VI. Egypt in the Middle Ages. Stanley Lane-Poole.

RELIGION AND CONSCIENCE IN ANCIENT EGYPT. Illustrated. *Cr. 8vo.* 2s. 6d.

SYRIA AND EGYPT, FROM THE TELL EL AMARNA LETTERS. *Cr. 8vo.* 2s. 6d.

EGYPTIAN TALES. Translated from the Papyri. First Series, Ivth to xiith Dynasty. Illustrated. *Second Edition. Cr. 8vo.* 3s. 6d.

EGYPTIAN TALES. Translated from the Papyri. Second Series, xviiith to xixth Dynasty. Illustrated. *Second Edition. Cr. 8vo.* 3s. 6d.

EGYPTIAN DECORATIVE ART. Illustrated. *Cr. 8vo.* 3s. 6d.

Phelps (Ruth S.). SKIES ITALIAN: A Little Breviary for Travellers in Italy. *Fcap 8vo. Leather,* 5s. *net.*

Pollard (Alfred W.). SHAKESPEARE FOLIOS AND QUARTOS. A Study in the Bibliography of Shakespeare's Plays, 1594-1685. Illustrated. *Folio.* 21s. *net.*

Porter (G. R.). THE PROGRESS OF THE NATION. A New Edition. Edited by F. W. Hirst. *Demy 8vo.* 21s. *net.*

Power (J. O'Connor). THE MAKING OF AN ORATOR. *Cr. 8vo.* 6s.

Price (Eleanor C.). CARDINAL DE RICHELIEU. Illustrated. *Second Edition. Demy 8vo.* 10s. 6d. *net.*

Price (L. L.). A SHORT HISTORY OF POLITICAL ECONOMY IN ENGLAND FROM ADAM SMITH TO ARNOLD TOYNBEE. *Seventh Edition. Cr. 8vo.* 2s. 6d.

Pycraft (W. P.). A HISTORY OF BIRDS. Illustrated. *Demy 8vo.* 10s. 6d. *net.*

Rawlings (Gertrude B.). COINS AND HOW TO KNOW THEM. Illustrated. *Third Edition. Cr. 8vo.* 6s.

Regan (C. Tait). THE FRESHWATER FISHES OF THE BRITISH ISLES. Illustrated. *Cr. 8vo.* 6s.

Reid (Archdall). THE LAWS OF HEREDITY. *Second Edition. Demy 8vo.* 21s. *net.*

Robertson (C. Grant). SELECT STATUTES, CASES, AND DOCUMENTS, 1660-1832. *Second and Enlarged Edition. Demy 8vo.* 10s. 6d. *net.*

ENGLAND UNDER THE HANOVERIANS. Illustrated. *Second Edition. Demy 8vo.* 10s. 6d. *net.*

Roe (Fred). OLD OAK FURNITURE. Illustrated. *Second Edition. Demy 8vo.* 10s. 6d *net.*

Ross (F. W. Forbes). CANCER: The Problem of its Genesis and Treatment. *Demy 8vo.* 5s. *net.*

Ryan (P. F. W.). STUART LIFE AND MANNERS: A Social History. Illustrated. *Demy 8vo.* 10s. 6d. *net.*

*Ryley (A. Beresford). OLD PASTE. Illustrated. *Royal 8vo.* £2 2s. *net.*

St. Francis of Assisi. THE LITTLE FLOWERS OF THE GLORIOUS MESSER, AND OF HIS FRIARS. Done into English, with Notes by William Heywood. Illustrated. *Demy 8vo.* 5s. *net.*

'Saki' (H. H. Monro). REGINALD. *Third Edition. Fcap. 8vo.* 2s. 6d. *net.*

REGINALD IN RUSSIA. *Fcap. 8vo.* 2s. 6d. *net.*

Sandeman (G. A. C.). METTERNICH. Illustrated. *Demy 8vo.* 10s. 6d. *net.*

Schidrowitz (Philip). RUBBER. Illustrated. *Demy 8vo.* 10s. 6d. *net.*

Schloesser (H. H.). TRADE UNIONISM. *Cr. 8vo.* 2s. 6d.

General Literature

Selous (Edmund). TOMMY SMITH'S ANIMALS. Illustrated. *Twelfth Edition. Fcap. 8vo.* 2s. 6d.

TOMMY SMITH'S OTHER ANIMALS. Illustrated. *Sixth Edition. Fcap. 8vo.* 2s. 6d.

JACK'S INSECTS. Illustrated. *Cr. 8vo.* 6s.

Shakespeare (William).
THE FOUR FOLIOS, 1623; 1632; 1664; 1685. Each £4 4s. net, or a complete set, £12 12s. net.

THE POEMS OF WILLIAM SHAKESPEARE. With an Introduction and Notes by George Wyndham. *Demy 8vo. Buckram,* 10s. 6d.

Shelley (Percy Bysshe). THE POEMS OF PERCY BYSSHE SHELLEY. With an Introduction by A. Clutton-Brock and notes by C. D. Locock. *Two Volumes. Demy 8vo.* 21s. net.

Sladen (Douglas). SICILY. The New Winter Resort. Illustrated. *Second Edition. Cr. 8vo.* 5s. net.

Smith (Adam). THE WEALTH OF NATIONS. Edited by Edwin Cannan. *Two Volumes. Demy 8vo.* 21s. net.

Smith (G. F. Herbert). GEM-STONES AND THEIR DISTINCTIVE CHARACTERS. Illustrated. *Second Edition. Cr. 8vo.* 6s. net.

Snell (F. J.). A BOOK OF EXMOOR. Illustrated. *Cr. 8vo.* 6s.

THE CUSTOMS OF OLD ENGLAND. Illustrated. *Cr. 8vo.* 6s.

'Stancliffe.' GOLF DO'S AND DONT'S. *Fifth Edition. Fcap. 8vo.* 1s. net.

Stevenson (R. L.). THE LETTERS OF ROBERT LOUIS STEVENSON. Edited by Sir Sidney Colvin. *A New and Enlarged Edition in four volumes. Third Edition. Fcap. 8vo. Each* 5s. *Leather, each* 5s. net.

Stevenson (M. I.). FROM SARANAC TO THE MARQUESAS AND BEYOND. Being Letters written by Mrs. M. I. Stevenson during 1887-88. Illustrated. *Cr. 8vo.* 6s. net.

LETTERS FROM SAMOA, 1891-95. Edited and arranged by M. C. Balfour. Illustrated. *Second Edition. Cr. 8vo.* 6s. net.

Storr (Vernon F.). DEVELOPMENT AND DIVINE PURPOSE. *Cr. 8vo.* 5s. net.

Streatfeild (R. A.). MODERN MUSIC AND MUSICIANS. Illustrated. *Second Edition. Demy 8vo.* 7s. 6d. net.

Swanton (E. W.). FUNGI AND HOW TO KNOW THEM. Illustrated. *Cr. 8vo.* 6s. net.

BRITISH PLANT-GALLS. *Cr. 8vo.* 7s. 6d. net.

Symes (J. E.). THE FRENCH REVOLUTION. *Second Edition. Cr. 8vo.* 2s. 6d.

Tabor (Margaret E.). THE SAINTS IN ART. Illustrated. *Third Edition. Fcap. 8vo.* 3s. 6d. net.

Taylor (A. E.). ELEMENTS OF METAPHYSICS. *Second Edition. Demy 8vo.* 10s. 6d. net.

Taylor (Mrs. Basil) (Harriet Osgood). JAPANESE GARDENS. Illustrated. *Cr. 4to.* 21s. net.

Thibaudeau (A. C.). BONAPARTE AND THE CONSULATE. Translated and Edited by G. K. Fortescue. Illustrated. *Demy 8vo.* 10s. 6d. net.

Thomas (Edward). MAURICE MAETERLINCK. Illustrated. *Second Edition. Cr. 8vo.* 5s. net.

Thompson (Francis). SELECTED POEMS OF FRANCIS THOMPSON. With a Biographical Note by Wilfrid Meynell. With a Portrait in Photogravure. *Twentieth Thousand. Fcap. 8vo.* 5s. net.

Tileston (Mary W.). DAILY STRENGTH FOR DAILY NEEDS. *Twentieth Edition. Medium 16mo.* 2s. 6d. net. Also an edition in superior binding, 6s.

THE STRONGHOLD OF HOPE. *Medium 16mo.* 2s. 6d. net.

Toynbee (Paget). DANTE ALIGHIERI. His Life and Works. With 16 Illustrations. *Fourth and Enlarged Edition. Cr. 8vo.* 5s. net.

Trevelyan (G. M.). ENGLAND UNDER THE STUARTS. With Maps and Plans. *Fifth Edition. Demy 8vo.* 10s. 6d. net.

Triggs (H. Inigo). TOWN PLANNING: Past, Present, and Possible. Illustrated. *Second Edition. Wide Royal 8vo.* 15s. net.

Turner (Sir Alfred E.). SIXTY YEARS OF A SOLDIER'S LIFE. *Demy 8vo.* 12s. 6d. net.

Underhill (Evelyn). MYSTICISM. A Study in the Nature and Development of Man's Spiritual Consciousness. *Fourth Edition. Demy 8vo.* 15s. net.

Underwood (F. M.). UNITED ITALY. *Demy 8vo.* 10s. 6d. net.

Urwick (E. J.). A PHILOSOPHY OF SOCIAL PROGRESS. *Cr. 8vo.* 6s.

Vardon (Harry). HOW TO PLAY GOLF. Illustrated. *Fifth Edition. Cr. 8vo.* 5s. net.

Vaughan (Herbert M.). THE NAPLES RIVIERA. Illustrated. *Second Edition. Cr. 8vo.* 6s.

FLORENCE AND HER TREASURES. Illustrated. *Fcap. 8vo. Round Corners.* 5s. net.

Vernon (Hon. W. Warren). READINGS ON THE INFERNO OF DANTE. With an Introduction by the Rev. Dr. MOORE. *Two Volumes. Second Edition. Cr. 8vo.* 15s. net.

READINGS ON THE PURGATORIO OF DANTE. With an Introduction by the late DEAN CHURCH. *Two Volumes. Third Edition. Cr. 8vo.* 15s. net.

READINGS ON THE PARADISO OF DANTE. With an Introduction by the BISHOP OF RIPON. *Two Volumes. Second Edition. Cr. 8vo.* 15s. net.

Vickers (Kenneth H.). ENGLAND IN THE LATER MIDDLE AGES. *Demy 8vo.* 10s. 6d. net.

Wade (G. W. and J. H.). RAMBLES IN SOMERSET. Illustrated. *Cr. 8vo.* 6s.

Waddell (L. A.). LHASA AND ITS MYSTERIES. With a Record of the Expedition of 1903-1904. Illustrated. *Third and Cheaper Edition. Medium 8vo.* 7s. 6d. net.

Wagner (Richard). RICHARD WAGNER'S MUSIC DRAMAS. Interpretations, embodying Wagner's own explanations. By ALICE LEIGHTON CLEATHER and BASIL CRUMP. *Fcap. 8vo.* 2s. 6d. each.

THE RING OF THE NIBELUNG.
Fifth Edition.

LOHENGRIN AND PARSIFAL.
Second Edition, rewritten and enlarged.

TRISTAN AND ISOLDE.

TANNHÄUSER AND THE MASTERSINGERS OF NUREMBURG.

Waterhouse (Elizabeth). WITH THE SIMPLE-HEARTED. Little Homilies to Women in Country Places. *Third Edition. Small Pott 8vo.* 2s. net.

THE HOUSE BY THE CHERRY TREE. A Second Series of Little Homilies to Women in Country Places. *Small Pott 8vo.* 2s. net.

COMPANIONS OF THE WAY. Being Selections for Morning and Evening Reading. Chosen and arranged by ELIZABETH WATERHOUSE. *Large Cr. 8vo.* 5s. net.

THOUGHTS OF A TERTIARY. *Small Pott 8vo.* 1s. net.

VERSES. *Fcap. 8vo.* 2s. net.

Waters (W. G.). ITALIAN SCULPTORS AND SMITHS. Illustrated. *Cr. 8vo.* 7s. 6d. net.

Watt (Francis). EDINBURGH AND THE LOTHIANS. Illustrated. *Second Edition. Cr. 8vo.* 10s. 6d. net.

Wedmore (Sir Frederick). MEMORIES. *Second Edition. Demy 8vo.* 7s. 6d. net.

Weigall (Arthur E. P.). A GUIDE TO THE ANTIQUITIES OF UPPER EGYPT: FROM ABYDOS TO THE SUDAN FRONTIER. Illustrated. *Second Edition. Cr. 8vo.* 7s. 6d. net.

Wells (J.). OXFORD AND OXFORD LIFE. *Third Edition. Cr. 8vo.* 3s. 6d.

A SHORT HISTORY OF ROME. *Twelfth Edition.* With 3 Maps. *Cr. 8vo.* 3s. 6d.

Whitten (Wilfred). A LONDONER'S LONDON. Illustrated. *Second Edition. Cr. 8vo.* 5s. net.

Wilde (Oscar). THE WORKS OF OSCAR WILDE. *In Twelve Volumes. Fcap. 8vo.* 5s. net each volume.

I. LORD ARTHUR SAVILE'S CRIME AND THE PORTRAIT OF MR. W. H. II. THE DUCHESS OF PADUA. III. POEMS. IV. LADY WINDERMERE'S FAN. V. A WOMAN OF NO IMPORTANCE. VI. AN IDEAL HUSBAND. VII. THE IMPORTANCE OF BEING EARNEST. VIII. A HOUSE OF POMEGRANATES. IX. INTENTIONS. X. DE PROFUNDIS AND PRISON LETTERS. XI. ESSAYS. XII. SALOMÉ, A FLORENTINE TRAGEDY, and LA SAINTE COURTISANE.

Williams (H. Noel). A ROSE OF SAVOY: MARIE ADÉLAÏDE OF SAVOY, DUCHESSE DE BOURGOGNE, MOTHER OF LOUIS XV. Illustrated. *Second Edition. Demy 8vo.* 15s. net.

THE FASCINATING DUC DE RICHELIEU: LOUIS FRANÇOIS ARMAND DU PLESSIS (1696-1788). Illustrated. *Demy 8vo.* 15s. net.

A PRINCESS OF ADVENTURE: MARIE CAROLINE, DUCHESSE DE BERRY (1798-1870). Illustrated. *Demy 8vo.* 15s. net.

THE LOVE AFFAIRS OF THE CONDÉS (1530-1740). Illustrated. *Demy 8vo.* 15s. net.

Wood (Sir Evelyn). FROM MIDSHIPMAN TO FIELD-MARSHAL. Illustrated. *Fifth Edition. Demy 8vo. 7s. 6d. net. Also Fcap. 8vo. 1s. net.*
THE REVOLT IN HINDUSTAN (1857-59). Illustrated. *Second Edition. Cr. 8vo. 6s.*

Wood (W. Birkbeck) and Edmonds (Col. J. E.). A HISTORY OF THE CIVIL WAR IN THE UNITED STATES (1861-65). With an Introduction by SPENSER WILKINSON. With 24 Maps and Plans. *Third Edition. Demy 8vo. 12s. 6d. net.*

Wordsworth (W.). THE POEMS. With an Introduction and Notes by NOWELL C. SMITH. *In Three Volumes. Demy 8vo. 15s. net.*

Yeats (W. B.). A BOOK OF IRISH VERSE. *Third Edition. Cr. 8vo. 3s. 6d.*

PART II.—A SELECTION OF SERIES

Ancient Cities

General Editor, B. C. A. WINDLE

Cr. 8vo. 4s. 6d. net each volume

With Illustrations by E. H. NEW, and other Artists

BRISTOL. Alfred Harvey.
CANTERBURY. J. C. Cox.
CHESTER. B. C. A. Windle.
DUBLIN. S. A. O. Fitzpatrick.
EDINBURGH. M. G. Williamson.
LINCOLN. E. Mansel Sympson.
SHREWSBURY. T. Auden.
WELLS and GLASTONBURY. T. S. Holmes.

The Antiquary's Books

General Editor, J. CHARLES COX

Demy 8vo. 7s. 6d. net each volume

With Numerous Illustrations

ANCIENT PAINTED GLASS IN ENGLAND, THE. Philip Nelson.
ARCHÆOLOGY AND FALSE ANTIQUITIES. R. Munro.
BELLS OF ENGLAND, THE. Canon J. J. Raven. *Second Edition.*
BRASSES OF ENGLAND, THE. Herbert W. Macklin. *Third Edition.*
CELTIC ART IN PAGAN AND CHRISTIAN TIMES. J. Romilly Allen. *Second Edition.*
CASTLES AND WALLED TOWNS OF ENGLAND, THE. A. Harvey.
DOMESDAY INQUEST, THE. Adolphus Ballard.
ENGLISH CHURCH FURNITURE. J. C. Cox and A. Harvey. *Second Edition.*
ENGLISH COSTUME. From Prehistoric Times to the End of the Eighteenth Century. George Clinch.
ENGLISH MONASTIC LIFE. Abbot Gasquet. *Fourth Edition.*
ENGLISH SEALS. J. Harvey Bloom.
FOLK-LORE AS AN HISTORICAL SCIENCE. Sir G. L. Gomme.

METHUEN AND COMPANY LIMITED

The Antiquary's Books—*continued*

GILDS AND COMPANIES OF LONDON, THE. George Unwin.

MANOR AND MANORIAL RECORDS, THE. Nathaniel J. Hone. *Second Edition.*

MEDIÆVAL HOSPITALS OF ENGLAND, THE. Rotha Mary Clay.

OLD CHURCHWARDENS' ACCOUNTS. J. C. Cox.

OLD ENGLISH INSTRUMENTS OF MUSIC. F. W. Galpin. *Second Edition.*

OLD ENGLISH LIBRARIES. James Hutt.

OLD SERVICE BOOKS OF THE ENGLISH CHURCH. Christopher Wordsworth, and Henry Littlehales. *Second Edition.*

PARISH LIFE IN MEDIÆVAL ENGLAND. Abbot Gasquet. *Third Edition.*

PARISH REGISTERS OF ENGLAND, THE. J. C. Cox.

REMAINS OF THE PREHISTORIC AGE IN ENGLAND. B. C. A. Windle. *Second Edition.*

ROMAN ERA IN BRITAIN, THE. J. Ward.

ROMANO-BRITISH BUILDINGS AND EARTHWORKS. J. Ward.

ROYAL FORESTS OF ENGLAND, THE. J. C. Cox.

SHRINES OF BRITISH SAINTS. J. C. Wall.

The Arden Shakespeare.

Demy 8vo. 2s. 6d. net each volume

An edition of Shakespeare in Single Plays; each edited with a full Introduction, Textual Notes, and a Commentary at the foot of the page

ALL'S WELL THAT ENDS WELL.
ANTONY AND CLEOPATRA. *Second Edition.*
AS YOU LIKE IT.
CYMBELINE.
COMEDY OF ERRORS, THE.
HAMLET. *Third Edition.*
JULIUS CAESAR.
*KING HENRY IV. PT. I.
KING HENRY V.
KING HENRY VI. PT. I.
KING HENRY VI. PT. II.
KING HENRY VI. PT. III.
KING LEAR.
KING RICHARD II.
KING RICHARD III.
LIFE AND DEATH OF KING JOHN, THE.
LOVE'S LABOUR'S LOST.

MACBETH.
MEASURE FOR MEASURE.
MERCHANT OF VENICE, THE. *Second Edition.*
MERRY WIVES OF WINDSOR, THE.
MIDSUMMER NIGHT'S DREAM, A.
OTHELLO.
PERICLES.
ROMEO AND JULIET.
TAMING OF THE SHREW, THE.
TEMPEST, THE.
TIMON OF ATHENS.
TITUS ANDRONICUS.
TROILUS AND CRESSIDA.
TWO GENTLEMEN OF VERONA, THE.
TWELFTH NIGHT.
VENUS AND ADONIS.
WINTER'S TALE, THE.

Classics of Art

Edited by DR. J. H. W. LAING

With numerous Illustrations. Wide Royal 8vo

THE ART OF THE GREEKS. H. B. Walters. 12s. 6d. net.

THE ART OF THE ROMANS. H. B. Walters. 15s. net.

CHARDIN. H. E. A. Furst. 12s. 6d. net.

DONATELLO. Maud Cruttwell. 15s. net.

FLORENTINE SCULPTORS OF THE RENAISSANCE. Wilhelm Bode. Translated by Jessie Haynes. 12s. 6d. net.

GEORGE ROMNEY. Arthur B. Chamberlain. 12s. 6d. net.

GENERAL LITERATURE 15

Classics of Art—*continued*

GHIRLANDAIO. Gerald S. Davies. *Second Edition.* 10s. 6d.

MICHELANGELO. Gerald S. Davies. 12s. 6d. net.

RUBENS. Edward Dillon. 25s. net.

RAPHAEL. A. P. Oppé. 12s. 6d. net.

REMBRANDT'S ETCHINGS. A. M. Hind.

SIR THOMAS LAWRENCE. Sir Walter Armstrong. 21s. net.

TITIAN. Charles Ricketts. 15s. net.

TINTORETTO. Evelyn March Phillipps. 15s. net.

TURNER'S SKETCHES AND DRAWINGS. A. J. Finberg. 12s. 6d. net. *Second Edition.*

VELAZQUEZ. A. de Beruete. 10s. 6d. net.

The 'Complete' Series.

Fully Illustrated. Demy 8vo

THE COMPLETE ASSOCIATION FOOTBALLER. B. S. Evers and C. E. Hughes-Davies. 5s. net.

THE COMPLETE BILLIARD PLAYER. Charles Roberts. 10s. 6d. net.

THE COMPLETE COOK. Lilian Whitling. 7s. 6d. net.

THE COMPLETE CRICKETER. Albert E. Knight. 7s. 6d. net. *Second Edition.*

THE COMPLETE FOXHUNTER. Charles Richardson. 12s. 6d. net. *Second Edition.*

THE COMPLETE GOLFER. Harry Vardon. 10s. 6d. net. *Thirteenth Edition.*

THE COMPLETE HOCKEY-PLAYER. Eustace E. White. 5s. net. *Second Edition.*

THE COMPLETE HORSEMAN. W. Scarth Dixon. *Second Edition.* 10s. 6d. net.

THE COMPLETE LAWN TENNIS PLAYER. A. Wallis Myers. 10s. 6d. net. *Third Edition, Revised.*

THE COMPLETE MOTORIST. Filson Young. 12s. 6d. net. *New Edition (Seventh).*

THE COMPLETE MOUNTAINEER. G. D. Abraham. 15s. net. *Second Edition.*

THE COMPLETE OARSMAN. R. C. Lehmann. 10s. 6d. net.

THE COMPLETE PHOTOGRAPHER. R. Child Bayley. 10s. 6d. net. *Fourth Edition.*

THE COMPLETE RUGBY FOOTBALLER, ON THE NEW ZEALAND SYSTEM. D. Gallaher and W. J. Stead. 10s. 6d. net. *Second Edition.*

THE COMPLETE SHOT. G. T. Teasdale-Buckell. 12s. 6d. net. *Third Edition.*

THE COMPLETE SWIMMER. F. Sachs. 7s. 6d. net.

THE COMPLETE YACHTSMAN. B. Heckstall-Smith and E. du Boulay. *Second Edition.* 15s. net.

The Connoisseur's Library

With numerous Illustrations. Wide Royal 8vo. 25s. net each volume

ENGLISH FURNITURE. F. S. Robinson.

ENGLISH COLOURED BOOKS. Martin Hardie.

ETCHINGS. Sir F. Wedmore. *Second Edition.*

EUROPEAN ENAMELS. Henry H. Cunynghame.

GLASS. Edward Dillon.

GOLDSMITHS' AND SILVERSMITHS' WORK. Nelson Dawson. *Second Edition.*

ILLUMINATED MANUSCRIPTS. J. A. Herbert. *Second Edition.*

IVORIES. Alfred Maskell.

JEWELLERY. H. Clifford Smith. *Second Edition.*

MEZZOTINTS. Cyril Davenport.

MINIATURES. Dudley Heath.

PORCELAIN. Edward Dillon.

FINE BOOKS. A. W. Pollard.

SEALS. Walter de Gray Birch.

WOOD SCULPTURE. Alfred Maskell. *Second Edition.*

Handbooks of English Church History

Edited by J. H. BURN. *Crown 8vo. 2s. 6d. net each volume*

THE FOUNDATIONS OF THE ENGLISH CHURCH. J. H. Maude.

THE SAXON CHURCH AND THE NORMAN CONQUEST. C. T. Cruttwell.

THE MEDIÆVAL CHURCH AND THE PAPACY. A. C. Jennings.

THE REFORMATION PERIOD. Henry Gee.

THE STRUGGLE WITH PURITANISM. Bruce Blaxland.

THE CHURCH OF ENGLAND IN THE EIGHTEENTH CENTURY. Alfred Plummer.

Handbooks of Theology

THE DOCTRINE OF THE INCARNATION. R. L. Ottley. *Fifth Edition, Revised. Demy 8vo.* 12s. 6d.

A HISTORY OF EARLY CHRISTIAN DOCTRINE. J. F. Bethune-Baker. *Demy 8vo.* 10s. 6d.

AN INTRODUCTION TO THE HISTORY OF RELIGION. F. B. Jevons. *Fifth Edition. Demy 8vo.* 10s. 6d.

AN INTRODUCTION TO THE HISTORY OF THE CREEDS. A. E. Burn. *Demy 8vo.* 10s. 6d.

THE PHILOSOPHY OF RELIGION IN ENGLAND AND AMERICA. Alfred Caldecott. *Demy 8vo.* 10s. 6d.

THE XXXIX ARTICLES OF THE CHURCH OF ENGLAND. Edited by E. C. S. Gibson. *Seventh Edition. Demy 8vo.* 12s. 6d.

The 'Home Life' Series

Illustrated. Demy 8vo. 6s. to 10s. 6d. net

HOME LIFE IN AMERICA. Katherine G. Busbey. *Second Edition.*

HOME LIFE IN FRANCE. Miss Betham-Edwards. *Sixth Edition.*

HOME LIFE IN GERMANY. Mrs. A. Sidgwick. *Second Edition.*

HOME LIFE IN HOLLAND. D. S. Meldrum. *Second Edition.*

HOME LIFE IN ITALY. Lina Duff Gordon. *Second Edition.*

HOME LIFE IN NORWAY. H. K. Daniels. *Second Edition.*

HOME LIFE IN RUSSIA. A. S. Rappoport.

HOME LIFE IN SPAIN. S. L. Bensusan. *Second Edition.*

The Illustrated Pocket Library of Plain and Coloured Books

Fcap. 8vo. 3s. 6d. net each volume

WITH COLOURED ILLUSTRATIONS

THE LIFE AND DEATH OF JOHN MYTTON, ESQ. Nimrod. *Fifth Edition.*

THE LIFE OF A SPORTSMAN. Nimrod.

HANDLEY CROSS. R. S. Surtees. *Fourth Edition.*

MR. SPONGE'S SPORTING TOUR. R. S. Surtees. *Second Edition.*

JORROCKS'S JAUNTS AND JOLLITIES. R. S. Surtees. *Third Edition.*

ASK MAMMA. R. S. Surtees.

THE ANALYSIS OF THE HUNTING FIELD. R. S. Surtees.

THE TOUR OF DR. SYNTAX IN SEARCH OF THE PICTURESQUE. William Combe.

THE TOUR OF DR. SYNTAX IN SEARCH OF CONSOLATION. William Combe.

THE THIRD TOUR OF DR. SYNTAX IN SEARCH OF A WIFE. William Combe.

LIFE IN LONDON. Pierce Egan.

WITH PLAIN ILLUSTRATIONS

THE GRAVE: A Poem. Robert Blair.

ILLUSTRATIONS OF THE BOOK OF JOB. Invented and Engraved by William Blake.

Leaders of Religion

Edited by H. C. BEECHING. *With Portraits*

Crown 8vo. 2s. net each volume

CARDINAL NEWMAN. R. H. Hutton.

JOHN WESLEY. J. H. Overton.

BISHOP WILBERFORCE. G. W. Daniell.

CARDINAL MANNING. A. W. Hutton.

CHARLES SIMEON. H. C. G. Moule.

JOHN KNOX. F. MacCunn. *Second Edition.*

JOHN HOWE. R. F. Horton.

THOMAS KEN. F. A. Clarke.

GEORGE FOX, THE QUAKER. T. Hodgkin. *Third Edition.*

JOHN KEBLE. Walter Lock.

THOMAS CHALMERS. Mrs. Oliphant. *Second Edition.*

LANCELOT ANDREWES. R. L. Ottley. *Second Edition.*

AUGUSTINE OF CANTERBURY. E. L. Cutts.

WILLIAM LAUD. W. H. Hutton. *Fourth Edition.*

JOHN DONNE. Augustus Jessop.

THOMAS CRANMER. A. J. Mason.

LATIMER. R. M. Carlyle and A. J. Carlyle.

BISHOP BUTLER. W. A. Spooner.

The Library of Devotion

With Introductions and (where necessary) Notes

Small Pott 8vo, cloth, 2s.; leather, 2s. 6d. net each volume

THE CONFESSIONS OF ST. AUGUSTINE. *Eighth Edition.*

THE IMITATION OF CHRIST. *Sixth Edition.*

THE CHRISTIAN YEAR. *Fifth Edition.*

LYRA INNOCENTIUM. *Third Edition.*

THE TEMPLE. *Second Edition.*

A BOOK OF DEVOTIONS. *Second Edition.*

A SERIOUS CALL TO A DEVOUT AND HOLY LIFE. *Fifth Edition.*

A GUIDE TO ETERNITY.

THE INNER WAY. *Second Edition.*

ON THE LOVE OF GOD.

THE PSALMS OF DAVID.

LYRICA APOSTOLICA.

THE SONG OF SONGS.

THE THOUGHTS OF PASCAL. *Second Edition.*

A MANUAL OF CONSOLATION FROM THE SAINTS AND FATHERS.

DEVOTIONS FROM THE APOCRYPHA.

THE SPIRITUAL COMBAT.

THE DEVOTIONS OF ST. ANSELM.

BISHOP WILSON'S SACRA PRIVATA.

GRACE ABOUNDING TO THE CHIEF OF SINNERS.

LYRA SACRA. A Book of Sacred Verse. *Second Edition.*

A DAY BOOK FROM THE SAINTS AND FATHERS.

A LITTLE BOOK OF HEAVENLY WISDOM. A Selection from the English Mystics.

LIGHT, LIFE, and LOVE. A Selection from the German Mystics.

AN INTRODUCTION TO THE DEVOUT LIFE.

THE LITTLE FLOWERS OF THE GLORIOUS MESSER ST. FRANCIS AND HIS FRIARS.

DEATH AND IMMORTALITY.

THE SPIRITUAL GUIDE. *Second Edition.*

DEVOTIONS FOR EVERY DAY IN THE WEEK AND THE GREAT FESTIVALS.

PRECES PRIVATAE.

HORAE MYSTICAE. A Day Book from the Writings of Mystics and Many Nations.

Little Books on Art

With many Illustrations. Demy 16mo. 2s. 6d. net each volume

Each volume consists of about 200 pages, and contains from 30 to 40 Illustrations, including a Frontispiece in Photogravure

ALBRECHT DÜRER. L. J. Allen.
ARTS OF JAPAN, THE. E. Dillon. *Third Edition.*
BOOKPLATES. E. Almack.
BOTTICELLI. Mary L. Bonnor.
BURNE-JONES. F. de Lisle.
CELLINI. R. H. H. Cust.
CHRISTIAN SYMBOLISM. Mrs. H. Jenner.
CHRIST IN ART. Mrs. H. Jenner.
CLAUDE. E. Dillon.
CONSTABLE. H. W. Tompkins. *Second Edition.*
COROT. A. Pollard and E. Birnstingl.
*EARLY ENGLISH WATER-COLOUR. C. E. Hughes.
ENAMELS. Mrs. N. Dawson. *Second Edition.*
FREDERIC LEIGHTON. A. Corkran.
GEORGE ROMNEY. G. PASTON.
GREEK ART. H. B. Walters. *Fourth Edition.*
GREUZE AND BOUCHER. E. F. Pollard.
HOLBEIN. Mrs. G. Fortescue.
ILLUMINATED MANUSCRIPTS. J. W. Bradley.
JEWELLERY. C. Davenport. *Second Edition.*
JOHN HOPPNER. H. P. K. Skipton.
SIR JOSHUA REYNOLDS. J. Sime. *Second Edition.*
MILLET. N. Peacock. *Second Edition.*
MINIATURES. C. Davenport. *Second Edition.*
OUR LADY IN ART. Mrs. H. Jenner.
RAPHAEL. A. R. Dryhurst.
REMBRANDT. Mrs. E. A. Sharp.
RODIN. Muriel Ciolkowska.
TURNER. F. Tyrrell-Gill.
VANDYCK. M. G. Smallwood.
VELAZQUEZ. W. Wilberforce and A. R. Gilbert.
WATTS. R. E. D. Sketchley. *Second Edition.*

The Little Galleries

Demy 16mo. 2s. 6d. net each volume

Each volume contains 20 plates in Photogravure, together with a short outline of the life and work of the master to whom the book is devoted

A LITTLE GALLERY OF REYNOLDS.
A LITTLE GALLERY OF ROMNEY.
A LITTLE GALLERY OF HOPPNER.
A LITTLE GALLERY OF MILLAIS.

The Little Guides

With many Illustrations by E. H. NEW and other artists, and from photographs

Small Pott 8vo. Cloth, 2s. 6d. net; leather, 3s. 6d. net each volume

The main features of these Guides are (1) a handy and charming form; (2) illustrations from photographs and by well-known artists; (3) good plans and maps; (4) an adequate but compact presentation of everything that is interesting in the natural features, history, archæology, and architecture of the town or district treated

CAMBRIDGE AND ITS COLLEGES. A. H. Thompson. *Third Edition, Revised.*
CHANNEL ISLANDS, THE. E. E. Bicknell.
ENGLISH LAKES, THE. F. G. Brabant.
ISLE OF WIGHT, THE. G. Clinch.
LONDON. G. Clinch.
MALVERN COUNTRY, THE. B. C. A. Windle.
NORTH WALES. A. T. STORY.

General Literature

The Little Guides—continued

Oxford and its Colleges. J. Wells. *Ninth Edition.*

St. Paul's Cathedral. G. Clinch.

Shakespeare's Country. B. C. A. Windle. *Fifth Edition.*

South Wales. G. W. and J. H. Wade.

Westminster Abbey. G. E. Troutbeck. *Second Edition.*

Berkshire. F. G. Brabant.

Buckinghamshire. E. S. Roscoe.

Cheshire. W. M. Gallichan.

Cornwall. A. L. Salmon. *Second Edition.*

Derbyshire. J. C. Cox.

Devon. S. Baring-Gould. *Second Edition.*

Dorset. F. R. Heath. *Second Edition.*

Durham. J. E. Hodgkin.

Essex. J. C. Cox.

Hampshire. J. C. Cox. *Second Edition.*

Hertfordshire. H. W. Tompkins.

Kent. G. Clinch.

Kerry. C. P. Crane. *Second Edition.*

Leicestershire and Rutland. A. Harvey and V. B. Crowther-Beynon.

Middlesex. J. B. Firth.

Monmouthshire. G. W. Wade and J. H. Wade.

Norfolk. W. A. Dutt. *Second Edition Revised.*

Northamptonshire. W. Dry. *New and Revised Edition.*

Northumberland. J. E. Morris.

Nottinghamshire. L. Guilford.

Oxfordshire. F. G. Brabant.

Shropshire. J. E. Auden.

Somerset. G. W. and J. H. Wade. *Second Edition.*

Staffordshire. C. Masefield.

Suffolk. W. A. Dutt.

Surrey. J. C. Cox.

Sussex. F. G. Brabant. *Third Edition.*

Wiltshire. F. R. Heath.

Yorkshire, The East Riding. J. E. Morris.

Yorkshire, The North Riding. J. E. Morris.

Yorkshire, The West Riding. J. E. Morris. *Cloth, 3s. 6d. net; leather, 4s. 6d. net.*

Brittany. S. Baring-Gould.

Normandy. C. Scudamore.

Rome. C. G. Ellaby.

Sicily. F. H. Jackson.

The Little Library

With Introduction, Notes, and Photogravure Frontispieces

Small Pott 8vo. Each Volume, cloth, 1s. 6d. net

Anon. A LITTLE BOOK OF ENGLISH LYRICS. *Second Edition.*

Austen (Jane). PRIDE AND PREJUDICE. *Two Volumes.*
NORTHANGER ABBEY.

Bacon (Francis). THE ESSAYS OF LORD BACON.

Barham (R. H.). THE INGOLDSBY LEGENDS. *Two Volumes.*

Barnett (Annie). A LITTLE BOOK OF ENGLISH PROSE.

Beckford (William). THE HISTORY OF THE CALIPH VATHEK.

Blake (William). SELECTIONS FROM THE WORKS OF WILLIAM BLAKE.

Borrow (George). LAVENGRO. *Two Volumes.*
THE ROMANY RYE.

Browning (Robert). SELECTIONS FROM THE EARLY POEMS OF ROBERT BROWNING.

Canning (George). SELECTIONS FROM THE ANTI-JACOBIN: With some later Poems by George Canning.

Cowley (Abraham). THE ESSAYS OF ABRAHAM COWLEY.

METHUEN AND COMPANY LIMITED

The Little Library—*continued*

Crabbe (George). SELECTIONS FROM THE POEMS OF GEORGE CRABBE.

Craik (Mrs.). JOHN HALIFAX, GENTLEMAN. *Two Volumes.*

Crashaw (Richard). THE ENGLISH POEMS OF RICHARD CRASHAW.

Dante Alighieri. THE INFERNO OF DANTE. Translated by H. F. CARY.
THE PURGATORIO OF DANTE. Translated by H. F. CARY.
THE PARADISO OF DANTE. Translated by H. F. CARY.

Darley (George). SELECTIONS FROM THE POEMS OF GEORGE DARLEY.

Deane (A. C.). A LITTLE BOOK OF LIGHT VERSE.

Dickens (Charles). CHRISTMAS BOOKS. *Two Volumes.*

Ferrier (Susan). MARRIAGE. *Two Volumes.*
THE INHERITANCE. *Two Volumes.*

Gaskell (Mrs.). CRANFORD. *Second Edition.*

Hawthorne (Nathaniel). THE SCARLET LETTER.

Henderson (T. F.). A LITTLE BOOK OF SCOTTISH VERSE.

Kinglake (A. W.). EOTHEN. *Second Edition.*

Lamb (Charles). ELIA, AND THE LAST ESSAYS OF ELIA.

Locker (F.). LONDON LYRICS.

Marvell (Andrew). THE POEMS OF ANDREW MARVELL.

Milton (John). THE MINOR POEMS OF JOHN MILTON.

Moir (D. M.). MANSIE WAUCH.

Nichols (Bowyer). A LITTLE BOOK OF ENGLISH SONNETS.

Smith (Horace and James). REJECTED ADDRESSES.

Sterne (Laurence). A SENTIMENTAL JOURNEY.

Tennyson (Alfred, Lord). THE EARLY POEMS OF ALFRED, LORD TENNYSON.
IN MEMORIAM.
THE PRINCESS.
MAUD.

Thackeray (W. M.). VANITY FAIR *Three Volumes.*
PENDENNIS. *Three Volumes.*
HENRY ESMOND.
CHRISTMAS BOOKS.

Vaughan (Henry). THE POEMS OF HENRY VAUGHAN.

Waterhouse (Elizabeth). A LITTLE BOOK OF LIFE AND DEATH. *Thirteenth Edition.*

Wordsworth (W.). SELECTIONS FROM THE POEMS OF WILLIAM WORDSWORTH.

Wordsworth (W.) and Coleridge (S. T.). LYRICAL BALLADS. *Second Edition.*

The Little Quarto Shakespeare

Edited by W. J. CRAIG. With Introductions and Notes

Pott 16mo. In 40 Volumes. Leather, price 1s. net each volume.

Mahogany Revolving Book Case. 10s. net

Miniature Library

Demy 32mo. Leather, 1s. net each volume

EUPHRANOR: A Dialogue on Youth. Edward FitzGerald.

THE LIFE OF EDWARD, LORD HERBERT OF CHERBURY. Written by himself.

POLONIUS; or, Wise Saws and Modern Instances. Edward FitzGerald.

THE RUBÁIYÁT OF OMAR KHAYYÁM. Edward FitzGerald. *Fourth Edition.*

GENERAL LITERATURE 21

The New Library of Medicine

Edited by C. W. SALEEBY. *Demy 8vo*

CARE OF THE BODY, THE. F. Cavanagh. *Second Edition.* 7s. 6d. net.

CHILDREN OF THE NATION, THE. The Right Hon. Sir John Gorst. *Second Edition.* 7s. 6d. net.

CONTROL OF A SCOURGE; or, How Cancer is Curable, The. Chas. P. Childe. 7s. 6d. net.

DISEASES OF OCCUPATION. Sir Thos. Oliver. 10s. 6d. net. *Second Edition.*

DRINK PROBLEM, in its Medico-Sociological Aspects, The. Edited by T. N. Kelynack. 7s. 6d. net.

DRUGS AND THE DRUG HABIT. H. Sainsbury.

FUNCTIONAL NERVE DISEASES. A. T. Schofield. 7s. 6d. net.

HYGIENE OF MIND, THE. T. S. Clouston. *Sixth Edition.* 7s. 6d. net.

INFANT MORTALITY. Sir George Newman. 7s. 6d. net.

PREVENTION OF TUBERCULOSIS (CONSUMPTION), THE. Arthur Newsholme. 10s. 6d. net. *Second Edition.*

AIR AND HEALTH. Ronald C. Macfie. 7s. 6d. net. *Second Edition.*

The New Library of Music

Edited by ERNEST NEWMAN. *Illustrated. Demy 8vo. 7s. 6d. net*

BRAHMS. J. A. Fuller-Maitland. *Second Edition.*

HANDEL. R. A. Streatfeild. *Second Edition.*

HUGO WOLF. Ernest Newman.

Oxford Biographies

Illustrated. Fcap. 8vo. Each volume, cloth, 2s. 6d. *net; leather,* 3s. 6d. *net*

DANTE ALIGHIERI. Paget Toynbee. *Third Edition.*

GIROLAMO SAVONAROLA. E. L. S. Horsburgh. *Sixth Edition.*

JOHN HOWARD. E. C. S. Gibson.

ALFRED TENNYSON. A. C. Benson. *Second Edition.*

SIR WALTER RALEIGH. I. A. Taylor.

ERASMUS. E. F. H. Capey.

ROBERT BURNS. T. F. Henderson.

CHATHAM. A. S. McDowall.

FRANCIS OF ASSISI. Anna M. Stoddart.

CANNING. W. Alison Phillips.

BEACONSFIELD. Walter Sichel.

JOHANN WOLFGANG GOETHE. H. G. Atkins.

FRANÇOIS DE FÉNELON. Viscount St. Cyres.

Four Plays

Fcap. 8vo. 2s. *net*

THE HONEYMOON. A Comedy in Three Acts. Arnold Bennett. *Second Edition.*

THE GREAT ADVENTURE. A Play of Fancy in Four Acts. Arnold Bennett. *Second Edition.*

MILESTONES. Arnold Bennett and Edward Knoblauch. *Sixth Edition.*

KISMET. Edward Knoblauch. *Second Edition.*

The States of Italy

Edited by E. ARMSTRONG and R. LANGTON DOUGLAS

Illustrated. Demy 8vo

A HISTORY OF MILAN UNDER THE SFORZA. Cecilia M. Ady. 10s. 6d. net.

A HISTORY OF PERUGIA. W. Heywood. 12s. 6d. net.

A HISTORY OF VERONA. A. M. Allen. 12s. 6d. net.

The Westminster Commentaries

General Editor, WALTER LOCK

Demy 8vo

THE ACTS OF THE APOSTLES. Edited by R. B. Rackham. *Sixth Edition.* 10s. 6d.

THE FIRST EPISTLE OF PAUL THE APOSTLE TO THE CORINTHIANS. Edited by H. L. Goudge. *Third Edition.* 6s.

THE BOOK OF EXODUS. Edited by A. H. M'Neile. With a Map and 3 Plans. 10s. 6d.

THE BOOK OF EZEKIEL. Edited by H. A. Redpath. 10s. 6d.

THE BOOK OF GENESIS. Edited, with Introduction and Notes, by S. R. Driver. *Ninth Edition.* 10s. 6d.

ADDITIONS AND CORRECTIONS IN THE SEVENTH AND EIGHTH EDITIONS OF THE BOOK OF GENESIS. S. R. Driver. 1s.

THE BOOK OF THE PROPHET ISAIAH. Edited by G. W. Wade. 10s. 6d.

THE BOOK OF JOB. Edited by E. C. S. Gibson. *Second Edition.* 6s.

THE EPISTLE OF ST. JAMES. Edited, with Introduction and Notes, by R. J. Knowling. *Second Edition.* 6s.

The 'Young' Series

Illustrated. Crown 8vo

THE YOUNG BOTANIST. W. P. Westell and C. S. Cooper. 3s. 6d. *net.*

THE YOUNG CARPENTER. Cyril Hall. 5s.

THE YOUNG ELECTRICIAN. Hammond Hall. 5s.

THE YOUNG ENGINEER. Hammond Hall. *Third Edition.* 5s.

THE YOUNG NATURALIST. W. P. Westell. *Second Edition.* 6s.

THE YOUNG ORNITHOLOGIST. W. P. Westell. 5s.

Methuen's Shilling Library

Fcap. 8vo. 1s. *net*

BLUE BIRD, THE. Maurice Maeterlinck.

CONDITION OF ENGLAND, THE. G. F. G. Masterman.

DE PROFUNDIS. Oscar Wilde.

FROM MIDSHIPMAN TO FIELD-MARSHAL. Sir Evelyn Wood, F.M., V.C.

HILLS AND THE SEA. Hilaire Belloc.

*HUXLEY, THOMAS HENRY. P. Chalmers-Mitchell.

IDEAL HUSBAND, AN. Oscar Wilde.

INTENTIONS. Oscar Wilde.

JIMMY GLOVER, HIS BOOK. James M. Glover.

JOHN BOYES, KING OF THE WA-KIKUYU. John Boyes.

LADY WINDERMERE'S FAN. Oscar Wilde.

LETTERS FROM A SELF-MADE MERCHANT TO HIS SON. George Horace Lorimer.

LIFE OF JOHN RUSKIN, THE. W. G. Collingwood.

LIFE OF ROBERT LOUIS STEVENSON, THE. Graham Balfour.

LIFE OF TENNYSON, THE. A. C. Benson.

LITTLE OF EVERYTHING, A. E. V. Lucas.

LORD ARTHUR SAVILE'S CRIME. Oscar Wilde.

LORE OF THE HONEY-BEE, THE. Tickner Edwardes.

MAN AND THE UNIVERSE. Sir Oliver Lodge.

MARY MAGDALENE. Maurice Maeterlinck.

OLD COUNTRY LIFE. S. Baring-Gould.

PARISH CLERK, THE. P. H. Ditchfield.

SELECTED POEMS. Oscar Wilde.

SEVASTOPOL, AND OTHER STORIES. Leo Tolstoy.

TWO ADMIRALS. Admiral John Moresby.

UNDER FIVE REIGNS. Lady Dorothy Nevill.

VAILIMA LETTERS. Robert Louis Stevenson.

VICAR OF MORWENSTOW, THE. S. Baring-Gould.

Books for Travellers

Crown 8vo. 6s. *each*

Each volume contains a number of Illustrations in Colour

A Wanderer in Florence. E. V. Lucas.
A Wanderer in Paris. E. V. Lucas.
A Wanderer in Holland. E. V. Lucas.
A Wanderer in London. E. V. Lucas.
The Norfolk Broads. W. A. Dutt.
The New Forest. Horace G. Hutchinson.
Naples. Arthur H. Norway.
The Cities of Umbria. Edward Hutton.
The Cities of Spain. Edward Hutton.
The Cities of Lombardy. Edward Hutton.
Florence and Northern Tuscany, with Genoa. Edward Hutton.
Siena and Southern Tuscany. Edward Hutton.
Rome. Edward Hutton.
Venice and Venetia. Edward Hutton.
The Bretons at Home. F. M. Gostling.
The Land of Pardons (Brittany). Anatole Le Braz.
A Book of the Rhine. S. Baring-Gould.
The Naples Riviera. H. M. Vaughan.
Days in Cornwall. C. Lewis Hind.
Through East Anglia in a Motor Car. J. E. Vincent.
The Skirts of the Great City. Mrs A. G. Bell.
Round about Wiltshire. A. G. Bradley.
Scotland of To-day. T. F. Henderson and Francis Watt.
Norway and its Fjords. M. A. Wyllie.

Some Books on Art

The Armourer and his Craft. Charles ffoulkes. Illustrated. *Royal 4to.* £2 2s. *net.*

Art and Life. T. Sturge Moore. Illustrated. *Cr. 8vo.* 5s. *net.*

Aims and Ideals in Art. George Clausen. Illustrated. *Second Edition. Large Post 8vo.* 5s. *net.*

Six Lectures on Painting. George Clausen. Illustrated. *Third Edition. Large Post 8vo.* 3s. 6d. *net.*

Francesco Guardi, 1712-1793. G. A. Simonson. Illustrated. *Imperial 4to.* £2 2s. *net.*

Illustrations of the Book of Job. William Blake. *Quarto.* £1 1s. *net.*

John Lucas, Portrait Painter, 1828-1874. Arthur Lucas. Illustrated. *Imperial 4to.* £3 3s *net.*

Old Paste. A. Beresford Ryley. Illustrated. *Royal 4to.* £2 2s. *net.*

One Hundred Masterpieces of Painting. With an Introduction by R. C. Witt. Illustrated. *Second Edition. Demy 8vo.* 10s. 6d. *net.*

The British School. An Anecdotal Guide to the British Painters and Paintings in the National Gallery. E. V. Lucas. Illustrated. *Fcap. 8vo.* 2s. 6d. *net.*

One Hundred Masterpieces of Sculpture. With an Introduction by G. F. Hill. Illustrated. *Demy 8vo.* 10s. 6d. *net.*

A Romney Folio. With an Essay by A. B. Chamberlain. *Imperial Folio.* £15 15s. *net.*

The Saints in Art. Margaret E. Tabor. Illustrated. *Second Edition. Fcap. 8vo.* 3s. 6d. *net.*

Schools of Painting. Mary Innes. Illustrated. *Cr. 8vo.* 5s. *net.*

Celtic Art in Pagan and Christian Times. J. R. Allen. Illustrated. *Second Edition. Demy 8vo.* 7s. 6d, *net.*

'Classics of Art.' See page 14.

'The Connoisseur's Library.' See page 15.

'Little Books on Art.' See page 18.

'The Little Galleries.' See page 18.

Some Books on Italy

ETRURIA AND MODERN TUSCANY, OLD. Mary L. Cameron. Illustrated. *Second Edition.* *Cr. 8vo.* 6s. *net.*

FLORENCE: Her History and Art to the Fall of the Republic. F. A. Hyett. *Demy 8vo.* 7s. 6d. *net.*

FLORENCE, A WANDERER IN. E. V. Lucas. Illustrated. *Fourth Edition.* *Cr. 8vo.* 6s.

FLORENCE AND HER TREASURES. H. M. Vaughan. Illustrated. *Fcap. 8vo.* 5s. *net.*

FLORENCE, COUNTRY WALKS ABOUT. Edward Hutton. Illustrated. *Second Edition.* *Fcap. 8vo.* 5s. *net.*

FLORENCE AND THE CITIES OF NORTHERN TUSCANY, WITH GENOA. Edward Hutton. Illustrated. *Second Edition.* *Cr. 8vo.* 6s.

LOMBARDY, THE CITIES OF. Edward Hutton. Illustrated. *Cr. 8vo.* 6s.

MILAN UNDER THE SFORZA, A HISTORY OF. Cecilia M. Ady. Illustrated. *Demy 8vo.* 10s. 6d. *net.*

NAPLES: Past and Present. A. H. Norway. Illustrated. *Third Edition.* *Cr. 8vo.* 6s.

NAPLES RIVIERA, THE. H. M. Vaughan. Illustrated. *Second Edition.* *Cr. 8vo.* 6s.

PERUGIA, A HISTORY OF. William Heywood. Illustrated. *Demy 8vo.* 12s. 6d. *net.*

ROME. Edward Hutton. Illustrated. *Third Edition.* *Cr. 8vo.* 6s.

ROME. C. G. Ellaby. Illustrated. *Small Pott 8vo.* Cloth, 2s. 6d. *net*; leather, 3s. 6d. *net.*

ROMAN PILGRIMAGE, A. R. E. Roberts. Illustrated. *Demy 8vo.* 10s. 6d. *net.*

SICILY. F. H. Jackson. Illustrated. *Small Pott 8vo.* Cloth, 2s. 6d. *net*; leather, 3s. 6d. *net.*

SICILY: The New Winter Resort. Douglas Sladen. Illustrated. *Second Edition.* *Cr. 8vo.* 5s. *net.*

SIENA AND SOUTHERN TUSCANY. Edward Hutton. Illustrated. *Second Edition.* *Cr. 8vo.* 6s.

TUSCANY, IN UNKNOWN. Edward Hutton. Illustrated. *Second Edition.* *Demy 8vo.* 7s. 6d. *net.*

UMBRIA, THE CITIES OF. Edward Hutton. Illustrated. *Fifth Edition.* *Cr. 8vo.* 6s.

VENICE AND VENETIA. Edward Hutton. Illustrated. *Cr. 8vo.* 6s.

VENICE ON FOOT. H. A. Douglas. Illustrated. *Second Edition.* *Fcap. 8vo.* 5s. *net.*

VENICE AND HER TREASURES. H. A. Douglas. Illustrated. *Fcap. 8vo.* 5s. *net.*

VERONA, A HISTORY OF. A. M. Allen. Illustrated. *Demy 8vo.* 12s. 6d. *net.*

DANTE AND HIS ITALY. Lonsdale Ragg. Illustrated. *Demy 8vo.* 12s. 6d. *net.*

DANTE ALIGHIERI: His Life and Works. Paget Toynbee. Illustrated. *Cr. 8vo.* 5s. *net.*

HOME LIFE IN ITALY. Lina Duff Gordon. Illustrated. *Third Edition.* *Demy 8vo.* 10s. 6d. *net.*

LAKES OF NORTHERN ITALY, THE. Richard Bagot. Illustrated. *Fcap. 8vo.* 5s. *net.*

LORENZO THE MAGNIFICENT. E. L. S. Horsburgh. Illustrated. *Second Edition.* *Demy 8vo.* 15s. *net.*

MEDICI POPES, THE. H. M. Vaughan. Illustrated. *Demy 8vo.* 15s. *net.*

ST. CATHERINE OF SIENA AND HER TIMES. By the Author of 'Mdlle. Mori.' Illustrated. *Second Edition.* *Demy 8vo.* 7s. 6d. *net.*

S. FRANCIS OF ASSISI, THE LIVES OF. Brother Thomas of Celano. *Cr. 8vo.* 5s. *net.*

SAVONAROLA, GIROLAMO. E. L. S. Horsburgh. Illustrated. *Cr. 8vo.* 5s. *net.*

SHELLEY AND HIS FRIENDS IN ITALY. Helen R. Angeli. Illustrated. *Demy 8vo.* 10s. 6d. *net.*

SKIES ITALIAN: A Little Breviary for Travellers in Italy. Ruth S. Phelps. *Fcap. 8vo.* 5s. *net.*

UNITED ITALY. F. M. Underwood. *Demy 8vo.* 10s. 6d. *net.*

WOMAN IN ITALY. W. Boulting. Illustrated. *Demy 8vo.* 10s. 6d. *net.*

Part III.—A Selection of Works of Fiction

Albanesi (E. Maria). SUSANNAH AND ONE OTHER. *Fourth Edition. Cr. 8vo. 6s.*
THE BROWN EYES OF MARY. *Third Edition. Cr. 8vo. 6s.*
I KNOW A MAIDEN. *Third Edition. Cr. 8vo. 6s.*
THE INVINCIBLE AMELIA; OR, THE POLITE ADVENTURESS. *Third Edition. Cr. 8vo. 3s. 6d.*
THE GLAD HEART. *Fifth Edition. Cr. 8vo. 6s.*
OLIVIA MARY. *Third Edition. Cr. 8vo. 6s.*
THE BELOVED ENEMY. *Second Edition. Cr. 8vo. 6s.*

Bagot (Richard). A ROMAN MYSTERY. *Third Edition Cr. 8vo. 6s.*
THE PASSPORT. *Fourth Edition. Cr. 8vo. 6s.*
ANTHONY CUTHBERT. *Fourth Edition. Cr. 8vo. 6s.*
LOVE'S PROXY. *Cr. 8vo. 6s.*
DONNA DIANA. *Second Edition. Cr. 8vo. 6s.*
CASTING OF NETS. *Twelfth Edition. Cr. 8vo. 6s.*
THE HOUSE OF SERRAVALLE. *Third Edition. Cr. 8vo. 6s.*
DARNELEY PLACE. *Second Edition. Cr. 8vo. 6s.*

Bailey (H. C.). STORM AND TREASURE. *Third Edition. Cr. 8vo. 6s.*
THE LONELY QUEEN. *Third Edition. Cr. 8vo. 6s.*

Baring-Gould (S.). IN THE ROAR OF THE SEA. *Eighth Edition. Cr. 8vo. 6s.*
MARGERY OF QUETHER. *Second Edition. Cr. 8vo. 6s.*
THE QUEEN OF LOVE. *Fifth Edition. Cr. 8vo. 6s.*
JACQUETTA. *Third Edition. Cr. 8vo. 6s.*
KITTY ALONE. *Fifth Edition. Cr. 8vo. 6s.*
NOÉMI. Illustrated. *Fourth Edition. Cr. 8vo. 6s.*
THE BROOM-SQUIRE. Illustrated. *Fifth Edition. Cr. 8vo. 6s.*
DARTMOOR IDYLLS. *Cr. 8vo. 6s.*
BLADYS OF THE STEWPONEY. Illustrated. *Second Edition. Cr. 8vo. 6s.*
PABO THE PRIEST. *Cr. 8vo. 6s.*
WINEFRED. Illustrated. *Second Edition. Cr. 8vo. 6s.*
ROYAL GEORGIE. Illustrated. *Cr. 8vo. 6s.*
IN DEWISLAND. *Second Edition. Cr. 8vo. 6s.*
MRS. CURGENVEN OF CURGENVEN. *Fifth Edition. Cr. 8vo. 6s.*

Barr (Robert). IN THE MIDST OF ALARMS. *Third Edition. Cr. 8vo. 6s.*
THE COUNTESS TEKLA. *Fifth Edition. Cr. 8vo. 6s.*
THE MUTABLE MANY. *Third Edition. Cr. 8vo. 6s.*

Begbie (Harold). THE CURIOUS AND DIVERTING ADVENTURES OF SIR JOHN SPARROW, BART.; OR, THE PROGRESS OF AN OPEN MIND. *Second Edition. Cr. 8vo. 6s.*

Belloc (H.). EMMANUEL BURDEN, MERCHANT. Illustrated. *Second Edition. Cr. 8vo. 6s.*
A CHANGE IN THE CABINET. *Third Edition. Cr. 8vo. 6s.*

Bennett (Arnold). CLAYHANGER. *Eleventh Edition. Cr. 8vo. 6s.*
THE CARD. *Ninth Edition. Cr. 8vo. 6s.*
HILDA LESSWAYS. *Seventh Edition. Cr. 8vo. 6s.*
BURIED ALIVE. *Third Edition. Cr. 8vo. 6s.*
A MAN FROM THE NORTH. *Third Edition. Cr. 8vo. 6s.*
THE MATADOR OF THE FIVE TOWNS. *Second Edition. Cr. 8vo. 6s.*

Benson (E. F.). DODO: A DETAIL OF THE DAY *Sixteenth Edition. Cr. 8vo. 6s.*

Birmingham (George A.). SPANISH GOLD. *Sixth Edition. Cr. 8vo. 6s.*
THE SEARCH PARTY. *Sixth Edition. Cr. 8vo. 6s.*
LALAGE'S LOVERS. *Third Edition. Cr. 8vo. 6s.*
THE ADVENTURES OF DR. WHITTY. *Fourth Edition. Cr. 8vo. 6s.*

METHUEN AND COMPANY LIMITED

Bowen (Marjorie). I WILL MAINTAIN. *Eighth Edition. Cr. 8vo. 6s.*
DEFENDER OF THE FAITH. *Sixth Edition. Cr. 8vo. 6s.*
A KNIGHT OF SPAIN. *Third Edition. Cr. 8vo. 6s.*
THE QUEST OF GLORY. *Third Edition. Cr. 8vo. 6s.*
GOD AND THE KING. *Fifth Edition. Cr. 8vo. 6s.*

Clifford (Mrs. W. K.). THE GETTING WELL OF DOROTHY. Illustrated. *Third Edition. Cr. 8vo. 3s. 6d.*

Conrad (Joseph). THE SECRET AGENT: A SIMPLE TALE. *Fourth Edition. Cr. 8vo. 6s.*
A SET OF SIX. *Fourth Edition. Cr. 8vo. 6s.*
UNDER WESTERN EYES. *Second Edition. Cr. 8vo. 6s.*

Conyers (Dorothea). SALLY. *Fourth Edition. Cr. 8vo. 6s.*

Corelli (Marie). A ROMANCE OF TWO WORLDS. *Thirty-Second Edition. Cr. 8vo. 6s.*
VENDETTA; OR, THE STORY OF ONE FORGOTTEN. *Thirtieth Edition. Cr. 8vo. 6s.*
THELMA: A NORWEGIAN PRINCESS. *Forty-third Edition. Cr. 8vo. 6s.*
ARDATH: THE STORY OF A DEAD SELF. *Twenty-first Edition. Cr. 8vo. 6s.*
THE SOUL OF LILITH. *Seventeenth Edition. Cr. 8vo. 6s.*
WORMWOOD: A DRAMA OF PARIS. *Nineteenth Edition. Cr. 8vo. 6s.*
BARABBAS: A DREAM OF THE WORLD'S TRAGEDY. *Forty-sixth Edition. Cr. 8vo. 6s.*
THE SORROWS OF SATAN. *Fifty-seventh Edition. Cr. 8vo. 6s.*
THE MASTER-CHRISTIAN. *Fourteenth Edition. 179th Thousand. Cr. 8vo. 6s.*
TEMPORAL POWER: A STUDY IN SUPREMACY. *Second Edition. 150th Thousand. Cr. 8vo. 6s.*
GOD'S GOOD MAN: A SIMPLE LOVE STORY. *Sixteenth Edition. 154th Thousand. Cr. 8vo. 6s.*
HOLY ORDERS: THE TRAGEDY OF A QUIET LIFE. *Second Edition. 120th Thousand. Cr. 8vo. 6s.*
THE MIGHTY ATOM. *Twenty-ninth Edition. Cr. 8vo. 6s.*
BOY: A SKETCH. *Thirteenth Edition. Cr. 8vo. 6s.*
CAMEOS. *Fourteenth Edition. Cr. 8vo. 6s.*
THE LIFE EVERLASTING. *Sixth Edition. Cr. 8vo. 6s.*

Crockett (S. R.). LOCHINVAR. Illustrated. *Third Edition. Cr. 8vo. 6s.*
THE STANDARD BEARER. *Second Edition. Cr. 8vo. 6s.*

Croker (B. M.). THE OLD CANTONMENT. *Second Edition. Cr. 8vo. 6s.*
JOHANNA. *Second Edition. Cr. 8vo. 6s.*
THE HAPPY VALLEY. *Fourth Edition. Cr. 8vo. 6s.*
A NINE DAYS' WONDER. *Fourth Edition. Cr. 8vo. 6s.*
PEGGY OF THE BARTONS. *Seventh Edition. Cr. 8vo. 6s.*
ANGEL. *Fifth Edition. Cr. 8vo. 6s.*
KATHERINE THE ARROGANT. *Sixth Edition. Cr. 8vo. 6s.*
BABES IN THE WOOD. *Fourth Edition. Cr. 8vo. 6s.*

Doyle (Sir A. Conan). ROUND THE RED LAMP. *Twelfth Edition. Cr. 8vo. 6s.*

Drake (Maurice). WO$_2$. *Fifth Edition. Cr. 8vo. 6s.*

Fenn (G. Manville). SYD BELTON: THE BOY WHO WOULD NOT GO TO SEA. Illustrated. *Second Edition. Cr. 8vo. 3s. 6d.*

Findlater (J. H.). THE GREEN GRAVES OF BALGOWRIE. *Fifth Edition. Cr. 8vo. 6s.*
THE LADDER TO THE STARS. *Second Edition. Cr. 8vo. 6s.*

Findlater (Mary). A NARROW WAY. *Third Edition. Cr. 8vo. 6s.*
THE ROSE OF JOY. *Third Edition. Cr. 8vo. 6s.*
A BLIND BIRD'S NEST. Illustrated. *Second Edition. Cr. 8vo. 6s.*

Fry (B. and C. B.). A MOTHER'S SON. *Fifth Edition. Cr. 8vo. 6s.*

Harraden (Beatrice). IN VARYING MOODS. *Fourteenth Edition. Cr. 8vo. 6s.*
HILDA STRAFFORD and THE REMITTANCE MAN. *Twelfth Edition. Cr. 8vo. 6s.*
INTERPLAY. *Fifth Edition. Cr. 8vo. 6s.*

Hauptmann (Gerhart). THE FOOL IN CHRIST. *Cr. 8vo. 6s.*

FICTION

Hichens (Robert). THE PROPHET OF BERKELEY SQUARE. *Second Edition. Cr. 8vo.* 6s.

TONGUES OF CONSCIENCE. *Third Edition. Cr. 8vo.* 6s.

FELIX: THREE YEARS IN A LIFE. *Tenth Edition. Cr. 8vo.* 6s.

THE WOMAN WITH THE FAN. *Eighth Edition. Cr. 8vo.* 6s.

BYEWAYS. *Cr. 8vo.* 6s.

THE GARDEN OF ALLAH. *Twenty-second Edition. Cr. 8vo.* 6s.

THE BLACK SPANIEL. *Cr. 8vo.* 6s.

THE CALL OF THE BLOOD. *Eighth Edition. Cr. 8vo.* 6s.

BARBARY SHEEP. *Second Edition. Cr. 8vo.* 3s. 6d.

THE DWELLER ON THE THRESHOLD. *Cr. 8vo.* 6s.

Hope (Anthony). THE GOD IN THE CAR. *Eleventh Edition. Cr. 8vo.* 6s.

A CHANGE OF AIR. *Sixth Edition. Cr. 8vo.* 6s.

A MAN OF MARK. *Seventh Edition. Cr. 8vo.* 6s.

THE CHRONICLES OF COUNT ANTONIO. *Sixth Edition. Cr. 8vo.* 6s.

PHROSO. Illustrated. *Ninth Edition. Cr. 8vo.* 6s.

SIMON DALE. Illustrated. *Ninth Edition. Cr. 8vo.* 6s.

THE KING'S MIRROR. *Fifth Edition. Cr. 8vo.* 6s.

QUISANTÉ. *Fourth Edition. Cr. 8vo.* 6s.

THE DOLLY DIALOGUES. *Cr. 8vo.* 6s.

TALES OF TWO PEOPLE. *Third Edition. Cr. 8vo.* 6s.

A SERVANT OF THE PUBLIC. Illustrated. *Sixth Edition. Cr. 8vo.* 6s.

THE GREAT MISS DRIVER. *Fourth Edition. Cr. 8vo.* 6s.

MRS. MAXTON PROTESTS. *Third Edition. Cr. 8vo.* 6s.

Hutten (Baroness von). THE HALO. *Fifth Edition. Cr. 8vo.* 6s.

'The Inner Shrine' (Author of). THE WILD OLIVE. *Third Edition. Cr. 8vo.* 6s.

THE STREET CALLED STRAIGHT. *Fourth Edition. Cr. 8vo.* 6s.

Jacobs (W. W.). MANY CARGOES. *Thirty-third Edition. Cr. 8vo.* 3s. 6d. Also Illustrated in colour. *Demy 8vo.* 7s. 6d. net.

SEA URCHINS. *Seventeenth Edition. Cr. 8vo.* 3s. 6d.

A MASTER OF CRAFT. Illustrated *Tenth Edition. Cr. 8vo.* 3s. 6d.

LIGHT FREIGHTS. Illustrated. *Eleventh Edition. Cr. 8vo.* 3s. 6d.

THE SKIPPER'S WOOING. *Eleventh Edition. Cr. 8vo.* 3s. 6d.

AT SUNWICH PORT. Illustrated. *Tenth Edition. Cr. 8vo.* 3s. 6d.

DIALSTONE LANE. Illustrated. *Eighth Edition. Cr. 8vo.* 3s. 6d.

ODD CRAFT. Illustrated. *Fifth Edition. Cr. 8vo.* 3s. 6d.

THE LADY OF THE BARGE. Illustrated. *Ninth Edition. Cr. 8vo.* 3s. 6d.

SALTHAVEN. Illustrated. *Third Edition. Cr. 8vo.* 3s. 6d.

SAILORS' KNOTS. Illustrated. *Fifth Edition. Cr. 8vo.* 3s. 6d.

SHORT CRUISES. *Third Edition. Cr. 8vo.* 3s. 6d.

James (Henry). THE GOLDEN BOWL. *Third Edition. Cr. 8vo.* 6s.

Le Queux (William). THE HUNCHBACK OF WESTMINSTER. *Third Edition. Cr. 8vo.* 6s.

THE CLOSED BOOK. *Third Edition. Cr. 8vo.* 6s.

THE VALLEY OF THE SHADOW. Illustrated. *Third Edition. Cr. 8vo.* 6s.

BEHIND THE THRONE. *Third Edition. Cr. 8vo.* 6s.

London (Jack). WHITE FANG. *Ninth Edition. Cr. 8vo.* 6s.

Lowndes (Mrs. Belloc). THE CHINK IN THE ARMOUR. *Fourth Edition. Cr. 8vo.* 6s.

MARY PECHELL. *Second Edition. Cr. 8vo.* 6s.

STUDIES IN LOVE AND TERROR. *Second Edition. Cr. 8vo.* 6s.

Lucas (E. V.). LISTENER'S LURE: AN OBLIQUE NARRATION. *Ninth Edition. Fcap. 8vo.* 5s.

OVER BEMERTON'S: AN EASY-GOING CHRONICLE. *Tenth Edition. Fcap. 8vo.* 5s.

MR. INGLESIDE. *Ninth Edition. Fcap. 8vo.* 5s.

LONDON LAVENDER. *Sixth Edition. Cr. 8vo.* 6s.

Lyall (Edna). DERRICK VAUGHAN, NOVELIST. *44th Thousand. Cr. 8vo,* 3s. 6d.

METHUEN AND COMPANY LIMITED

Macnaughtan (S.). THE FORTUNE OF CHRISTINA M'NAB. *Sixth Edition. Cr. 8vo. 6s.*
PETER AND JANE. *Fourth Edition. Cr. 8vo. 6s.*

Malet (Lucas). A COUNSEL OF PERFECTION. *Second Edition. Cr. 8vo. 6s.*
COLONEL ENDERBY'S WIFE. *Sixth Edition. Cr. 8vo. 6s.*
THE HISTORY OF SIR RICHARD CALMADY: A ROMANCE. *Ninth Edition. Cr. 8vo. 6s.*
THE WAGES OF SIN. *Sixteenth Edition. Cr. 8vo. 6s.*
THE CARISSIMA. *Fifth Edition. Cr. 8vo. 6s.*
THE GATELESS BARRIER. *Fifth Edition. Cr. 8vo. 6s.*

Mason (A. E. W.). CLEMENTINA. Illustrated. *Eighth Edition. Cr. 8vo. 6s.*

Maxwell (W. B.). THE RAGGED MESSENGER. *Third Edition. Cr. 8vo. 6s.*
VIVIEN. *Twelfth Edition. Cr. 8vo. 6s.*
THE GUARDED FLAME. *Seventh Edition. Cr. 8vo. 6s.*
ODD LENGTHS. *Second Edition. Cr. 8vo. 6s.*
HILL RISE. *Fourth Edition. Cr. 8vo. 6s.*
THE COUNTESS OF MAYBURY: BETWEEN YOU AND I. *Fourth Edition. Cr. 8vo. 6s.*
THE REST CURE. *Fourth Edition. Cr. 8vo. 6s.*

Milne (A. A.). THE DAY'S PLAY. *Fourth Edition. Cr. 8vo. 6s.*
THE HOLIDAY ROUND. *Second Edition. Cr. 8vo. 6s.*

Montague (C. E.). A HIND LET LOOSE. *Third Edition. Cr. 8vo. 6s.*

Morrison (Arthur). TALES OF MEAN STREETS. *Seventh Edition. Cr. 8vo. 6s.*
A CHILD OF THE JAGO. *Sixth Edition. Cr. 8vo. 6s.*
THE HOLE IN THE WALL. *Fourth Edition. Cr. 8vo. 6s.*
DIVERS VANITIES. *Cr. 8vo. 6s.*

Ollivant (Alfred). OWD BOB, THE GREY DOG OF KENMUIR. With a Frontispiece. *Twelfth Edition. Cr. 8vo. 6s.*
THE TAMING OF JOHN BLUNT. *Second Edition. Cr. 8vo. 6s.*
THE ROYAL ROAD. *Second Edition. Cr. 8vo. 6s.*

Onions (Oliver). GOOD BOY SELDOM: A ROMANCE OF ADVERTISEMENT. *Second Edition. Cr. 8vo. 6s.*

Oppenheim (E. Phillips). MASTER OF MEN. *Fifth Edition. Cr. 8vo. 6s.*
THE MISSING DELORA. Illustrated. *Fourth Edition. Cr. 8vo. 6s.*

Orczy (Baroness). FIRE IN STUBBLE. *Fifth Edition. Cr. 8vo. 6s.*

Oxenham (John). A WEAVER OF WEBS. Illustrated. *Fifth Edition. Cr. 8vo. 6s.*
THE GATE OF THE DESERT. *Eighth Edition. Cr. 8vo. 6s.*
PROFIT AND LOSS. *Fourth Edition. Cr. 8vo. 6s.*
THE LONG ROAD. *Fourth Edition. Cr. 8vo. 6s.*
THE SONG OF HYACINTH, AND OTHER STORIES. *Second Edition. Cr. 8vo. 6s.*
MY LADY OF SHADOWS. *Fourth Edition. Cr. 8vo. 6s.*
LAURISTONS. *Fourth Edition. Cr. 8vo. 6s.*
THE COIL OF CARNE. *Sixth Edition. Cr. 8vo. 6s.*
THE QUEST OF THE GOLDEN ROSE. *Fourth Edition. Cr. 8vo. 6s.*
MARY ALL-ALONE. *Third Edition. Cr. 8vo. 6s.*

Parker (Gilbert). PIERRE AND HIS PEOPLE. *Seventh Edition. Cr. 8vo. 6s.*
MRS. FALCHION. *Fifth Edition. Cr. 8vo. 6s.*
THE TRANSLATION OF A SAVAGE. *Fourth Edition. Cr. 8vo. 6s.*
THE TRAIL OF THE SWORD. Illustrated. *Tenth Edition. Cr. 8vo. 6s.*
WHEN VALMOND CAME TO PONTIAC: THE STORY OF A LOST NAPOLEON. *Seventh Edition. Cr. 8vo. 6s.*
AN ADVENTURER OF THE NORTH: THE LAST ADVENTURES OF 'PRETTY PIERRE.' *Fifth Edition. Cr. 8vo. 6s.*
THE SEATS OF THE MIGHTY. Illustrated. *Nineteenth Edition. Cr. 8vo. 6s.*
THE BATTLE OF THE STRONG: A ROMANCE OF TWO KINGDOMS. Illustrated. *Seventh Edition. Cr. 8vo. 6s.*
THE POMP OF THE LAVILETTES. *Third Edition. Cr. 8vo. 3s. 6d.*
NORTHERN LIGHTS. *Fourth Edition. Cr. 8vo. 6s.*

Pasture (Mrs. Henry de la). THE TYRANT. *Fourth Edition. Cr. 8vo. 6s.*

FICTION

Pemberton (Max). THE FOOTSTEPS OF A THRONE. Illustrated. *Fourth Edition. Cr. 8vo. 6s.*

I CROWN THEE KING. Illustrated. *Cr. 8vo. 6s.*

LOVE THE HARVESTER: A STORY OF THE SHIRES. Illustrated. *Third Edition. Cr. 8vo. 3s. 6d.*

THE MYSTERY OF THE GREEN HEART. *Fifth Edition. Cr. 8vo. 6s.*

Perrin (Alice). THE CHARM. *Fifth Edition. Cr. 8vo. 6s.*

THE ANGLO-INDIANS. *Sixth Edition. Cr. 8vo. 6s.*

Phillpotts (Eden). LYING PROPHETS. *Third Edition. Cr. 8vo. 6s.*

CHILDREN OF THE MIST. *Sixth Edition. Cr. 8vo. 6s.*

THE HUMAN BOY. With a Frontispiece. *Seventh Edition. Cr. 8vo. 6s.*

SONS OF THE MORNING. *Second Edition. Cr. 8vo. 6s.*

THE RIVER. *Fourth Edition. Cr. 8vo. 6s.*

THE AMERICAN PRISONER. *Fourth Edition. Cr. 8vo. 6s.*

KNOCK AT A VENTURE. *Third Edition. Cr. 8vo. 6s.*

THE PORTREEVE. *Fourth Edition. Cr. 8vo. 6s.*

THE POACHER'S WIFE. *Second Edition. Cr. 8vo. 6s.*

THE STRIKING HOURS. *Second Edition. Cr. 8vo. 6s.*

DEMETER'S DAUGHTER. *Third Edition. Cr. 8vo. 6s.*

Pickthall (Marmaduke). SAÏD, THE FISHERMAN. *Eighth Edition. Cr. 8vo. 6s.*

'Q' (A. T. Quiller-Couch). THE MAYOR OF TROY. *Fourth Edition. Cr. 8vo. 6s.*

MERRY-GARDEN AND OTHER STORIES. *Cr. 8vo. 6s.*

MAJOR VIGOUREUX. *Third Edition. Cr. 8vo. 6s.*

Ridge (W. Pett). ERB. *Second Edition. Cr. 8vo. 6s.*

A SON OF THE STATE. *Third Edition. Cr. 8vo. 3s. 6d.*

A BREAKER OF LAWS. *A New Edition. Cr. 8vo. 3s. 6d.*

MRS. GALER'S BUSINESS. Illustrated. *Second Edition. Cr. 8vo. 6s.*

THE WICKHAMSES. *Fourth Edition. Cr. 8vo. 6s.*

SPLENDID BROTHER. *Fourth Edition. Cr. 8vo. 6s.*

NINE TO SIX-THIRTY. *Third Edition. Cr. 8vo. 6s.*

THANKS TO SANDERSON. *Second Edition. Cr. 8vo. 6s.*

DEVOTED SPARKES. *Second Edition. Cr. 8vo. 6s.*

Russell (W. Clark). MASTER ROCKAFELLAR'S VOYAGE. Illustrated. *Fourth Edition. Cr. 8vo. 3s. 6d.*

Sidgwick (Mrs. Alfred). THE KINSMAN. Illustrated. *Third Edition. Cr. 8vo. 6s.*

THE LANTERN-BEARERS. *Third Edition. Cr. 8vo. 6s.*

THE SEVERINS. *Sixth Edition. Cr. 8vo. 6s.*

ANTHEA'S GUEST. *Fourth Edition. Cr. 8vo. 6s.*

LAMORNA. *Third Edition. Cr. 8vo. 6s.*

Snaith (J. C.). THE PRINCIPAL GIRL. *Second Edition. Cr. 8vo. 6s.*

AN AFFAIR OF STATE. *Second Edition. Cr. 8vo. 6s.*

Somerville (E. Œ.) and Ross (Martin). DAN RUSSEL THE FOX. Illustrated. *Seventh Edition. Cr. 8vo. 6s.*

Thurston (E. Temple). MIRAGE. *Fourth Edition. Cr. 8vo. 6s.*

Watson (H. B. Marriott). ALISE OF ASTRA. *Third Edition. Cr. 8vo. 6s.*

THE BIG FISH. *Third Edition. Cr. 8vo. 6s.*

Webling (Peggy). THE STORY OF VIRGINIA PERFECT. *Third Edition. Cr. 8vo. 6s.*

THE SPIRIT OF MIRTH. *Sixth Edition. Cr. 8vo. 6s.*

FELIX CHRISTIE. *Third Edition. Cr. 8vo. 6s.*

THE PEARL STRINGER. *Second Edition. Cr. 8vo. 6s.*

Weyman (Stanley). UNDER THE RED ROBE. Illustrated. *Twenty-third Edition. Cr. 8vo. 6s.*

Whitby (Beatrice). ROSAMUND. *Second Edition. Cr. 8vo. 6s.*

Williamson (C. N. and A. M.). THE LIGHTNING CONDUCTOR: The Strange Adventures of a Motor Car. Illustrated. *Twenty-first Edition. Cr. 8vo. 6s. Also Cr. 8vo. 1s. net.*

THE PRINCESS PASSES: A ROMANCE OF A MOTOR. Illustrated. *Ninth Edition.* Cr. 8vo. 6s. net.

LADY BETTY ACROSS THE WATER. *Eleventh Edition.* Cr. 8vo. 6s.

THE BOTOR CHAPERON. Illustrated. *Eighth Edition.* Cr. 8vo. 6s.

THE CAR OF DESTINY. Illustrated. *Seventh Edition.* Cr. 8vo. 6s.

MY FRIEND THE CHAUFFEUR. Illustrated. *Twelfth Edition.* Cr. 8vo. 6s.

SCARLET RUNNER. Illustrated. *Third Edition.* Cr. 8vo. 6s.

SET IN SILVER. Illustrated. *Fourth Edition.* Cr. 8vo. 6s.

LORD LOVELAND DISCOVERS AMERICA. *Second Edition.* Cr. 8vo. 6s.

THE GOLDEN SILENCE. *Sixth Edition.* Cr. 8vo. 6s.

THE GUESTS OF HERCULES. *Third Edition.* Cr. 8vo. 6s.

THE HEATHER MOON. *Fifth Edition.* Cr. 8vo. 6s.

THE LOVE PIRATE. *Second Edition.* Cr. 8vo. 6s.

Wyllarde (Dolf). THE PATHWAY OF THE PIONEER (Nous Autres). *Sixth Edition.* Cr. 8vo. 6s.

Methuen's Two-Shilling Novels

Crown 8vo. 2s. net

BOTOR CHAPERON, THE. C. N. and A. M. Williamson.

CALL OF THE BLOOD, THE. Robert Hichens.

CARD, THE. Arnold Bennett.

CLEMENTINA. A. E. W. Mason.

COLONEL ENDERBY'S WIFE. Lucas Malet.

FELIX. Robert Hichens.

GATE OF THE DESERT, THE. John Oxenham.

MY FRIEND THE CHAUFFEUR. C. N. and A. M. Williamson.

MYSTERY OF THE GREEN HEART, THE. Max Pemberton.

OLD GORGON GRAHAM. G. H. Lorimer.

PRINCESS VIRGINIA, THE. C. N and A. M. Williamson.

SEARCH PARTY, THE. G. A. Birmingham.

SEATS OF THE MIGHTY, THE. Sir Gilbert Parker.

SERVANT OF THE PUBLIC, A. Anthony Hope.

SET IN SILVER. C. N. and A. M. Williamson.

SEVERINS, THE. Mrs. Alfred Sidgwick.

SIR RICHARD CALMADY. Lucas Malet.

VIVIEN. W. B. Maxwell.

Books for Boys and Girls

Illustrated. Crown 8vo. 3s. 6d.

GETTING WELL OF DOROTHY, THE. Mrs. W. K. Clifford.

GIRL OF THE PEOPLE, A. L. T. Meade.

HEPSY GIPSY. L. T. Meade. 2s. 6d.

HONOURABLE MISS, THE. L. T. Meade.

MASTER ROCKAFELLAR'S VOYAGE. W. Clark Russell.

ONLY A GUARD-ROOM DOG. Edith E. Cuthell.

RED GRANGE, THE. Mrs. Molesworth.

SYD BELTON: The Boy who would not go to Sea. G. Manville Fenn.

THERE WAS ONCE A PRINCE. Mrs. M. E. Mann.

Methuen's Shilling Novels

Fcap. 8vo. 1s. net

ANNA OF THE FIVE TOWNS. Arnold Bennett.
BARBARY SHEEP. Robert Hichens.
CHARM, THE. Alice Perrin.
DAN RUSSEL THE FOX. E. Œ. Somerville and Martin Ross.
DEMON, THE. C. N. and A. M. Williamson.
FIRE IN STUBBLE. Baroness Orczy.
GUARDED FLAME, THE. W. B. Maxwell.
HILL RISE. W. B. Maxwell.
JANE. Marie Corelli.
JOSEPH IN JEOPARDY. Frank Danby.
LADY BETTY ACROSS THE WATER. C. N. and A. M. Williamson.
LIGHT FREIGHTS. W. W. Jacobs.
LONG ROAD, THE. John Oxenham.
MIGHTY ATOM, THE. Marie Corelli.
MIRAGE. E. Temple Thurston.
MISSING DELORA, THE. E. Phillips Oppenheim.
ROUND THE RED LAMP. Sir A. Conan Doyle.
SAÏD, THE FISHERMAN. Marmaduke Pickthall.
SECRET WOMAN, THE. Eden Phillpotts.
SEVERINS, THE. Mrs. Alfred Sidgwick.
SPANISH GOLD. G. A. Birmingham.
SPLENDID BROTHER. W. Pett Ridge.
TALES OF MEAN STREETS. Arthur Morrison.
HALO, THE. Baroness von Hutten.
TYRANT, THE. Mrs. Henry de la Pasture.
UNDER THE RED ROSE. Stanley J. Weyman.
VIRGINIA PERFECT. Peggy Webling.
WOMAN WITH THE FAN, THE. Robert Hichens.

Methuen's Sevenpenny Novels

Fcap. 8vo. 7d. net

ANGEL. B. M. CROKER.

PRINCE RUPERT THE BUCCANEER. C. J. CUTCLIFFE HYNE.

I CROWN THEE KING. MAX PEMBERTON.

THE BROOM SQUIRE. S. BARING-GOULD.

LONE PINE. R. B. TOWNSHEND.

THE SIGN OF THE SPIDER. BERTRAM MITFORD.

MASTER OF MEN. E. PHILLIPS OPPENHEIM.

THE POMP OF THE LAVILETTES. Sir GILBERT PARKER.

THE HUMAN BOY. EDEN PHILLPOTTS.

BY STROKE OF SWORD. ANDREW BALFOUR.

Printed by MORRISON & GIBB LIMITED, *Edinburgh*